CONTENTS

PREAMBLE

Age Concern has endeavoured over the years to be at the forefront of debate on issues of importance to older people. Sometimes this has meant that we address matters which others hesitate to take on board so soon. We feel it is important, however, to ensure that full and frank information and advice are available to those who seek to know more on a particular subject to meet their own needs or to help those they love and care for at a personal level or through their work.

It is in this vein that we decided to publish this important book. We hope it will contribute in a sensitive way towards helping sufferers and older carers of people who are HIV positive or who think they may be vulnerable to AIDS and help to prevent or alleviate the difficulties and distress many experience.

For obvious reasons, certain sections of the book have had to be written in an explicit manner. We trust that readers will understand this and not be offended by any of the content.

Sally Greengross
Director General
Age Concern England

HIV&AIDS
and older people

Tara Kaufmann

30130504005668

Dedication

To my grandparents, Felix and Ruth.

Published by Age Concern England
1268 London Road
London SW16 4ER

Editor Gillian Clarke
Design and typesetting Eugenie Dodd Typographics
Copy preparation Vinnette Marshall
Printed in Great Britain by Bell and Bain Ltd, Glasgow
Cover photograph by Sunil Gupta

A catalogue record for this book is available
from the British Library.

ISBN 0–86242–181–0

ABOUT THE AUTHOR

Tara Kaufmann is a freelance writer whose previous publications include books on unplanned pregnancy and gay politics; she is currently writing a book on modern marriage. She has worked for a number of charities covering issues such as reproductive health, drug and alcohol misuse, employment rights and mental health. Tara has also worked for Age Concern London and is the author of their report *A Crisis of Silence: HIV, AIDS and Older People.*

ACKNOWLEDGEMENTS

Acknowledgements are due to the groundbreaking work carried out by the Age Concern in London Working Group on HIV and AIDS. Particular thanks go to Paula Jones, Alistair Beattie and Liz Barker from Age Concern London.

Debby Klein generously shared her skills as a counsellor, writer and HIV trainer, providing valuable advice on both style and content. Thanks are also offered to Eva Heymann, counsellor at the Terrence Higgins Trust, and Dr Adam Lawrence for their helpful comments on the book.

Warm thanks go to all the older people who have shared their experiences of HIV and AIDS, especially Kingsley Slocombe-Wood, Betty Feldman, Reg and Doreen Langbridge, Reg Martin and Joe Humble.

The tables in Chapter 6 are adapted with kind permission from *Caring in a Crisis: what to do and who to turn to* by Marina Lewycka (ACE Books).

Additional research was carried out by Ros Powell.

1.
What have HIV and AIDS got to do with you?

"AIDS is everyone's problem."

"AIDS doesn't discriminate."

"AIDS is an equal opportunity disease."

How often have you heard these slogans, and what did you understand them to mean? That you don't have to be gay to be affected by HIV and AIDS? That you don't have to be male? That you don't have to be white?

But before you had reason to pick up this book, did it occur to you that AIDS was not just an issue for the young?

As you are reading this book, you presumably have some awareness or concern about HIV and AIDS. You may be an older person yourself, or perhaps you are personally or professionally concerned about a particular older person, or about older people in general. You probably know more about this issue than the average person. But do you know just how extensive the impact of HIV and AIDS on older people has been?

By the end of December 1994 there were 22,645 reported cases of HIV, and 10,272 of AIDS, in England and Wales. Of these, 1,342 people with HIV were aged 50 and over, and 1,086 had been diagnosed with AIDS. For reasons we will discuss later, the real total may be much higher.

This means that over one in ten people with AIDS are aged over 50. (If you think of the 'celebrity cases' of people with AIDS, you'll find many men in later life, such as Denholm Elliot, Rock Hudson, Tony Richardson and Rudolf Nureyev.) As the population ages, and an increasingly large proportion of people become over pensionable age, so we can expect the average age of people with HIV or AIDS to rise.

What is particularly interesting about the official statistics is the similarity in patterns of HIV infection across all adult age groups. Among both older and younger people in the United Kingdom, more men than women have been infected with HIV. The major route of transmission is sexual contact – mostly sex between men but an ever-growing proportion from heterosexual sex. This is largely due to historical accident, because the gay community was infected by HIV early on; however, the number and proportion of cases of heterosexual transmission are rising.

Before 1985, when donated blood started to be screened, a number of older people were infected with HIV through blood transfusions or donated blood products (older people are major recipients of donated blood). Injecting drug use has not been implicated in HIV transmission in this age group, though undoubtedly there are older people who do inject drugs.

Yet the myth that AIDS is a disease of youth is strong – whether you hold 'sympathetic' stereotypes of people with AIDS as young and full of promise, or more negative views of AIDS as a consequence of 'too much' sex or sex with the 'wrong' people.

This is partly because AIDS is often perceived as a disease of the modern era. It gets talked about as though it somehow represents and typifies everything that is wrong with the late twentieth century. Sometimes people talk with misty-eyed nostalgia about sex before the shadow of AIDS as if it were an age of innocence, forgetting the very real problems of unplanned pregnancy, sexually transmitted diseases such as syphilis and gonorrhoea, and ruined reputations. The fact is that sex has never been 'safe', and modern morality did not 'cause' HIV and AIDS.

But the myth that AIDS is a young people's problem persists, mainly because it is a disease associated with sex – and older people aren't supposed to have sex. Younger people – and, surprisingly, older people too – often think that the elderly are 'past all that', that it is somehow inappropriate or ridiculous or even disgusting for older people to seek and give sexual pleasure.

The denial of sex

Contrary to what many younger people think, there is no automatic decline in sexual appetite or behaviour as we get older. Older people can and do have active sex lives. They may have less sex than younger people (though studies suggest that even young people have less sex than is often supposed) but this is usually less to do with lack of desire than with poor health, loss of a partner, social and emotional problems, or as a side effect of certain medications.

Older people often share this belief that sex is for the young: in fact, they may feel deeply ashamed of having sexual impulses 'at their age'. They may face very real prejudices and even punishment for sexual behaviour. We've all heard older men who are interested in sex being called 'dirty old men', while the idea that older women may like sex is considered almost disgusting.

This prejudice is reflected in institutional practices, such as the discouragement of sexual behaviour in care homes. Although residential care staff are increasingly likely to accept the right of established heterosexual couples to share a bed, more casual relationships – or same-sex relationships – are usually frowned upon. Older sex is seen as embarrassing and undignified: of course, this view only encourages older people to feel guilty and abnormal, and spoils their chances of developing and maintaining normal sexual relationships.

The need for caring and intimacy begins very early in human development, and it does not disappear as we get older. In fact, it may become more important in later life, as friends and family move away or die, as it becomes more difficult to go out and start new relationships, and as loneliness becomes increasingly common. It is very important for older people to be able to be physically and emotionally close to others.

One 20-year study looked at how sexual behaviour changed over time among a group of people aged between 60 and 94. They found that interest in sex was very common, and that it tended to stay strong over time. What did change as people got older was the opportunity for translating this interest into action. The reasons for this varied: women tended to reserve sex for their husbands, and so to give up sex after widowhood, whereas men's sexual activity was more commonly undermined by declining health and the side effects of medications.

Masters and Johnson (in their well known book published in 1970) found that men and women in generally good health were physically able to have a satisfying sex life well into their 70s and beyond, and that those who retained sexual vigour and sexual interest throughout their youth and middle age would continue to do so into old age. The most common cause of sexual dysfunction in the older man is not physiological, they concluded, but due to other factors such as performance anxiety. Both sexes are strongly influenced in their sexual behaviour by their own attitudes to it and its importance in their lives.

It is mainly in Western culture that sexuality in later life is considered so unusual. And this prejudice is at least partly to blame for the spread of HIV and AIDS among the elderly because it has prevented older people being offered or asking for information about protection against HIV.

Not infected, but affected

There are other ways in which older people feel the impact of HIV and AIDS on their lives. One of the results of the unfavourable press given to people with HIV or AIDS in the United Kingdom has been the portrayal of them as big city deviants, unattached to families or communities in which 'people like us' live. But over 20,000 people are known to have HIV: most of them will have family and friends who in turn feel the impact of HIV on their lives. They may be older people who are nursing sons or daughters, grandparents of children orphaned by AIDS, spouses or brothers or sisters.

Many people with AIDS will 'go home' to elderly parents when they get very ill. There are also older people caring for younger friends, relatives or even lodgers with HIV. HIV and AIDS affect people of all ages, cultures and walks of life, with no regard for whether they think they 'deserve' it or are expecting it.

You may be the main carer for someone with HIV or AIDS, coping with all the additional roles and stresses facing carers. Or you may not be living with the loved one with HIV, but desperately concerned to help in whatever way you can – and not sure how to do that.

If you have only recently become aware that a family member has HIV or AIDS, you will want to find out the truth about the infection and how it is transmitted. Grandparents may be anxious that there might be some risk to their grandchildren if, for example, they kiss a relative (or family friend) who has HIV. Myths and half-truths abound regarding the infection and how it may be passed on, and can cause needless anxiety for anyone who, until now, has seen no reason to sift fact from fiction. You will be looking for reassurance and guidance.

Maybe you just need some general information about HIV and AIDS and how to reduce your risk of contracting it. Perhaps you are or intend to be sexually active, and would like to know how to do so safely. Or you could be worried that past experience has put you at risk of HIV, and want to put your mind at rest.

Perhaps you are already doing your bit to help people with HIV and AIDS. Charities such as the Terrence Higgins Trust and London Lighthouse report that many of their 'buddies' and other volunteers are older people, with time on their hands and a lifetime of experience to contribute.

How this book can help

This book aims to provide basic information and advice for older people who are directly or indirectly affected by HIV or AIDS. It will also be useful for anyone who is concerned about an older person infected or affected by HIV or AIDS.

Chapter 2 contains essential information about HIV and AIDS: what the terms mean; how HIV is transmitted and diagnosed; and the symptoms and progression of HIV disease. There is also important advice about how people can protect themselves and those they love from HIV infection – even if you do not think you could ever be in a position to become infected with HIV, this section is worth reading so that you can pass the information on to others, if need be.

Chapter 3 is aimed at older people who are the family, friends, lovers and/or carers of someone with HIV infection. It also contains sections that will be useful to older people with HIV themselves, such as advice on whom to tell and when, and common relationship problems. There are two case studies of older people: Betty, whose son died with AIDS, and Kingsley, who is a carer for someone with AIDS.

Chapter 4 is intended mainly for older people who are themselves infected with HIV – although, again, it contains information of interest and value to everyone. It explores in more detail how older people get infected with HIV, and the impact infection has on their physical and emotional health. Two older men with HIV – Joe and

Reg – tell their stories in this chapter, along with Elizabeth, an older woman with AIDS.

In Chapter 5 there is further discussion of the day-to-day issues to be faced by people if HIV or AIDS is part of their life, including emotional and relationship problems. Chapter 6 covers some of the practical issues, and gives guidance on the help available. It can be read right through, or different sections can be dipped into as they become relevant.

Finally, there is a comprehensive section of Useful Addresses, to signpost sources of further advice and practical support.

2.
What people need to know about HIV and AIDS

In the early 1980s, a strange new disease started surfacing in the American gay community. Previously healthy, fit young men were falling ill and dying for reasons that couldn't yet be explained. It was thought that the appearance of this new virus might be rooted in some aspect of the gay lifestyle, and in 1981 it was labelled GRID – short for 'Gay Related Immune Deficiency'. This was the disease now known as 'AIDS'.

It wasn't long before other groups of people started showing signs of HIV infection – injecting drug users, haemophiliacs, people who'd had blood transfusions – and it was realised that *anyone* could contract the condition. Scientists soon dropped the term 'GRID', and it has been known for many years that there is nothing intrinsic in the gay lifestyle that 'causes' AIDS. Unfortunately, the first media reports about HIV and AIDS unleashed a wave of bigotry against gay men, and many people choose to continue thinking of AIDS as 'the gay plague'.

These days, there is still a lot that is not known about this disease – particularly in terms of its treatment and possible cure – but a lot more is understood about its transmission and its impact on people's health. The terms now used to talk about this disease are HIV and AIDS. Often these two words are spoken in the same breath as though they are the same thing, or one of them is used instead of the other as though they were interchangeable. In fact, they are two distinct terms, and the distinction is important.

HIV is short for Human Immunodeficiency Virus. A virus is a micro-organism that can survive only inside the cells of other living creatures. HIV damages the immune system, weakening the body's defences against infection and disease. When people become infected with HIV, they produce antibodies to the virus which can be detected in their blood: these people are said to be HIV positive (HIV+). Many people infected with HIV have no symptoms at all and they look and feel perfectly well. Others may suffer problems such as swollen glands or fever – with varying degrees of severity. Current medical opinion – although this has been challenged – is that most people who have HIV will go on to develop AIDS, even though this may be months, years or over a decade after infection.

AIDS stands for Acquired Immune Deficiency Syndrome. When a person is diagnosed as having AIDS, it means that they have developed one or more of the infections or cancers which have been shown to be related to an immune system that has been permanently damaged by HIV infection. Two of the most common of these are a particular form of pneumonia called PCP (for '*Pneumocystis carinii* pneumonia') and the skin cancer Kaposi's sarcoma.

Even when someone has AIDS, ill health may be sporadic, and they may continue to live and work normally for much of the time. It is the cancers and the 'opportunistic' infections, not AIDS itself, that cause death. At the time of writing, AIDS is considered fatal, although people may live for many years after diagnosis.

The definitions of HIV and AIDS are sometimes confusing, and do not reflect the widely differing patterns of HIV infection that affect individuals. As a result, many agencies now talk more generally of *HIV illness* or *HIV disease* to refer to all medical conditions and illnesses related to infection with HIV.

How is HIV spread?

There is perhaps more fear and misunderstanding about the transmission of HIV than about any disease since leprosy. Many people think that HIV is highly contagious and can be passed on through swimming pools, toilet seats or coffee cups. Others see HIV as a disease that affects 'only' homosexuals, or drug users, or (in Europe) Africans or (in Asia) Europeans.

In fact, HIV is *not* contagious and cannot be 'caught' from general social contact such as shaking hands, sharing crockery, using toilets, sneezing or kissing. There is absolutely no reason to isolate or reject people with HIV or AIDS: many people have been deeply hurt through such rejection at a time when they most need companionship and support.

Anyone can contract HIV under certain conditions: fortunately, a lot is known about what those conditions are and how to avoid them. HIV is a relatively fragile virus when encountered in everyday work or social situations (it is easily killed by bleach, disinfectant, and exposure to water or air). It can, however, be transmitted through getting infected semen, vaginal fluids or blood into the bloodstream. The most common ways in which people become infected with HIV are:

- unprotected penetrative sex (vaginal or anal) with someone who has HIV infection;
- receiving infected blood through sharing needles or syringes with someone who is infected with the virus;
- from an infected pregnant woman to her child, either during pregnancy or at birth, or possibly through breastfeeding;
- receiving infected blood products or a blood transfusion. This risk has been virtually eliminated in Western countries since the introduction of screening for donated blood and heat-treating of blood products in 1985.

In the United Kingdom, most of the people who have been tested positive for HIV have been gay men or injecting drug users. This is only because they were the *first* groups of people to be affected – in other countries heterosexuals make up the majority of those with HIV. So there is no reason to suppose that someone who is not gay is 'safe': many of the people most at risk will be those who assume that HIV infection is nothing to do with them. Widespread complacency and misplaced social condemnation are major contributors to the spread of HIV.

Another unhelpful myth has been the assumption that HIV is 'caused' by promiscuity, and therefore that monogamy is the best protection against it. The trouble is that, although it may be easy to look at other people's sex lives and label them as 'sleeping around', very few individuals can see their own relationships in those terms. There are also many people who have contracted HIV in long-term relationships or with their first sexual partners – and many others who have very busy sex lives but who practise safer sex and so will be less likely to get HIV. The virus does not know – and certainly does not care – whether people are married to the person they are sleeping with, whether they are in love, whether they even know each other's names.

At the end of the day, the number of people someone sleeps with is only one factor to take into account when calculating the risk from HIV. A person could sleep with hundreds of people without risk from HIV, if none of them had the virus. Or that individual could be unlucky enough to contract HIV from their very first sexual encounter, or from a partner with whom they are in a long-term, committed relationship. Not only does this mean that everyone has a responsibility to think about safer sex and other ways of reducing the risk of HIV in their lives, it also means everyone has a responsibility not to judge or make assumptions about those who have contracted HIV or AIDS.

Diagnosing HIV and AIDS

People with HIV infection can live healthily for many years, completely unaware of their condition. That is why the statistics on HIV and AIDS are likely to under-estimate the true scale of the problem, and why – ideally – everybody should think through the implications of HIV for their lives, and reach an informed decision about whether they should adopt safer sex to protect themselves against infection.

Many people do not know they are infected with HIV until they develop symptoms. These symptoms may be attributed to other medical conditions and there is some suggestion that older people, and women in particular, are vulnerable to misdiagnosis by doctors because HIV is not thought of as a possibility.

Other people discover their situation by taking the HIV antibody test, often incorrectly referred to as the 'AIDS test'. This is not actually a test for AIDS at all, but a blood test to detect the antibodies that are produced in response to HIV. A negative result means that antibodies to HIV have not been found, and so HIV infection is unlikely. However, it can take three months, or sometimes longer, from the time of infection for antibodies to show up in a blood test, so a negative result is reliable only if the individual hasn't been at risk in the last three months. (Many people repeat the test after three months to make sure of this.) A positive result means that antibodies to HIV have been found. This does not mean that the person has AIDS; but it does mean that they have HIV infection which can be passed on to others, even though they may look and feel well.

A positive test result can be emotionally devastating and sometimes leads to practical problems such as difficulty obtaining life insurance or a mortgage: a negative result can lead to a false sense of security and low motivation to practise safer sex. Either way, it is important that each individual reaches their own decision whether or not to be tested, and that they are offered specialist counselling by a trained adviser.

GPs can arrange an HIV test, but they won't necessarily have any special training on HIV, and the result goes on to the patient's medical records. Most people prefer to go to a genito-urinary medicine (GUM) clinic – these are also known by the terms 'special clinic', 'STD clinic' or 'VD clinic'. GUM clinics have an image problem, and many people are embarrassed or reluctant to attend them. But people from every walk of life go to GUM clinics, and the staff there are trained to be respectful and sensitive to their clients' feelings. They will offer specialist counselling both before and after the HIV test, and a visit there is totally confidential and will never end up on the GP's medical records. The easiest way to find the nearest GUM clinic is to look in the *Yellow Pages*, or just ring your local hospital.

What are the symptoms of HIV and AIDS?

Any list of symptoms associated with AIDS will include a number of conditions that people may suffer from every year: tiredness, swollen glands, weight loss, chills, diarrhoea, thrush and dry cough. Even when very seriously ill, people with AIDS often have cancers or diseases (such as tuberculosis or pneumonia) that also afflict people who are not HIV positive. No doctor can diagnose AIDS from any symptom without knowing the results of an HIV antibody test – and neither can anyone else. So assumptions should never be made about HIV status from any set of symptoms – it's simply not reliable.

AIDS has been called 'the great pretender', because it often mimics symptoms that are commonly found in that group of people anyway. Women, for example, tend to experience symptoms of AIDS in ways that are different from men – with gynaecological problems such as discharges, cervical irregularities or cancer of the womb or cervix. There is some evidence that older people have symptoms of AIDS in ways that are rather different from the pattern of disease among younger people. More information can be found in Chapter 5.

How are HIV and AIDS treated?

At present there is no cure for HIV or AIDS and no vaccine against infection by HIV. There is a great deal of research going on into drug treatments to boost the immune system and slow the progression of HIV, and progress is being made in these areas.

Medical treatment of the illnesses associated with HIV is advancing all the time, and conventional medicine has a lot to offer in the control and treatment of the many and varied illnesses and infections someone with HIV may suffer over a number of years. So it certainly makes sense for specialist medical advice to be sought as soon as a diagnosis of HIV is made.

Many people with HIV also make use of a range of complementary medicines and holistic treatments, including massage, acupuncture, homoeopathy, visualisation and special diets. Although they are unlikely to cure HIV infection, they are very helpful in making people feel better.

People with HIV or AIDS can also do a lot to help themselves, particularly by taking good care of their immune systems. This means eating a nutritious diet, high in protein and calories; resting and sleeping well; avoiding cold and damp living conditions; and reducing excessive stress and exhaustion. This sounds easier than it sometimes is, of course, particularly when someone lives in poor housing or on a very low income. More information on this is available in Chapter 6.

Protecting against HIV infection

Everyone needs to know how to protect themselves from HIV infection, whatever their age or lifestyle. As you are reading this book, you are probably already concerned about HIV, and treating it seriously. However, you may still feel that this section isn't important for you.

There are, though, good reasons for learning about safer sex. One is that you may find yourself in a position to offer information and advice to others who are at risk. Perhaps you have a grandchild who is worried and confused about AIDS; perhaps a friend has just started a new relationship and is too embarrassed to ask anyone else for advice: wouldn't you like to be able to help?

Maybe you feel you're unlikely to start a new relationship at your time of life. Maybe you're in a long-term monogamous relationship, and you're sure neither of you has been unfaithful to each other. Maybe you absolutely *know* – because of disinclination, disease or infirmity – that sex is not on the cards for you. Or maybe you're thinking, 'OK, there's a chance I might start a sexual relationship with someone who is HIV positive. But frankly I'm more likely to die from heart disease or cancer or getting knocked down in the High Street, so I think I'll take my chances.'

If that's your choice then fine – we all make choices every day about the risks we are prepared to take, and in the end the decision must be yours. But it is a good idea to make *informed* decisions, and you really should know about the risks and how you can reduce them before you decide whether or not you want to take preventative action.

Another reason for getting informed is to stop yourself worrying unnecessarily. AIDS helplines report that a large number of their calls are from the 'worried well' – people whose risk of contracting HIV is low, but who none the less are eaten up with worry about it. This kind of obsession is usually caused by a combination of misinformation and sexual guilt. Being informed about HIV and AIDS is *not* an admission that you are at risk: it *is* a way of equipping yourself to make informed decisions about what kind of risks you are prepared to run in your own life.

Safer sex

Most HIV transmission is through sex. The good news is that there are practical steps which anyone can take to protect themselves without having to give up sex or stop having fun in bed. Practising safer sex means that it is not necessary to rely on the other person to be honest about their sexual history, nor does it have to be assumed that they have not got the virus when they may have been at risk. It's a sensible procedure which, with practice, becomes second nature – like wearing a seat belt in the car.

Most safer sex is common sense if it is remembered that a person is at risk only if the HIV virus can pass from infected body fluids into their bloodstream. Three body fluids contain enough of the virus to pose a risk: blood, semen and vaginal fluid. There are a number of ways of making love that will not put someone at risk because they don't involve exchange of body fluids. Unprotected anal or vaginal sex is risky because it could let infected body fluids inside their body – this is the most common way of getting infected with HIV – so it makes sense to wear a condom. Here are the steps any individual can take to protect themselves.

- A condom should always be used when starting a new relationship or if there is any reason to suppose that either partner has been exposed to HIV. Condoms (also once called french letters or rubber johnnies) can be bought across the counter in any chemist's shop, or in most supermarkets, or mail order – there are advertisements in the back of many newspapers and magazines. The condoms should carry a British Standard kitemark, and be of the right strength: extra-strong condoms are available for anal sex. The condom must always be used within its sell-by date, and it shouldn't be carried around in a back pocket or somewhere that heat can damage it. Care should also be taken not to damage condoms with sharp objects such as keys or jewellery.

- If a lubricant is used, it must be water-based (K-Y Jelly is the best-known brand). Oil-based lubricants such as Vaseline petroleum jelly, massage oil or butter will rot the condom.

- Many men feel nervous about putting condoms on correctly: this may be particularly nerve-racking if it has been many years since they last wore a condom, or if they have problems gaining or sustaining an erection. It is a good idea to try a 'dress rehearsal': practise putting a condom on and masturbating with one on when alone.

- When putting on a condom the penis should be erect. The teat is held between thumb and forefinger to expel the air (trapped air inside a condom can make it split). Care must be taken not to tear the condom on fingernails or rings.

- The penis should be withdrawn immediately after ejaculation. This way the condom is less likely to leak.

- If the condom breaks or comes off, there is no need to panic. It's obviously not ideal, but it doesn't mean that the partner will automatically get the virus. Even if the person is HIV positive, the partner's chance of contracting the virus through any one episode of unprotected sex has been calculated at about one in fifty. A ripped condom must be kept in perspective.

- People can enjoy using condoms. The ones available today really are very different from the thick condoms of yesteryear, and come in different textures, colours and flavours.

There may be reasons why people don't want to use condoms: perhaps their religion prohibits the use of contraceptives, or maybe they don't have penetrative sex because of worries about sustaining an erection. There are lots of other ways in which to give and receive sexual pleasure; plenty of books give advice and ideas on this – they can be found in mainstream bookshops.

Oral sex is considered fairly safe so long as the mouth is healthy. There is a higher risk of transmission if there are cuts, sores or infections in the mouth or throat. It is still a lot less risky than vaginal or anal sex, but if someone is worried they can buy (flavoured) condoms. For oral sex with a woman, it is possible to use a condom that has been cut open, or a dental dam (these are thin latex sheets you can buy from some dental suppliers).

Other examples of safer sex practices include kissing, hugging and cuddling, massage, masturbating each other (touching or coming on the outside of the body), fantasy and sex toys (but if both partners want to penetrate each other with the same sex toy, they must be sure to wash it or use a condom on it). Of course, not all these ways of making love may appeal to everyone, and no one should do anything in bed that makes them feel bad about themselves or about the person they are with.

Difficulties with safer sex

People may say, 'That sounds easy in principle, but the practice is quite different'. They are right, it is different. Older people may find adopting safer sex particularly difficult, as many will have grown up in a time and place where sexual activity, or even discussion of sexual behaviour, has been regarded as 'dirty' or 'secret'. This may make it very hard for them to talk openly and honestly about sex with their partner. It may also make them reluctant to experiment with new ways of having sex.

For someone in a long-term relationship, introducing safer sex can be seen as a vote of no confidence in their partner's fidelity, or as an implicit admission that they have been 'playing around' themselves.

An older man who has or has had sex with men will have grown up in a society where homosexual activity was not only frowned upon but actually illegal. As a consequence he may not be openly gay, and so may not have access to specialist safer sex information for gay men. He may even be married, and worried that he is putting his wife as well as himself at risk because of fear that introducing safer sex into his marriage will raise too many awkward questions.

There are no easy answers to these situations – at the end of the day it is up to each person to decide how many changes they want to make in their life, and what difficulties they want to take on. But before they give it all up as impossible, they should seek advice and talk it over with a trained counsellor or a friend. Unfortunately, older people do not often come into contact with major sources of health education and advice about HIV, such as family planning clinics. But there are other sources of help, such as the National AIDS

Helpline, or one of the counselling schemes run by Age Concern around the country. A number of sources of help and advice are listed in the Useful Addresses section.

Safer drug use

Illicit drug use is relatively rare among older people. But this does mean that if someone *is* involved with drug misuse, they are particularly likely to feel very isolated and alone.

It is more likely, however, that an older person will be worried by the drug use of a child or grandchild. Having a drug user in the family can be very painful and destructive for all involved. Parents and grandparents often feel helpless in the face of a child's drug habit, and terrified for the future. As with HIV infection, it is easy to panic and assume that death is imminent if the drug use is not stopped immediately. It may be far harder to work with the drug user to maintain calm, non-chaotic drug use and to maximise good health. Parents and grandparents in this situation can obtain a lot of support from local counselling and self-help groups. Getting practical information on safer drug use from a specialist HIV agency such as Mainliners, as well as emotional support and advice from a service for the families of drug users such as Adfam National, will help both the drug user and their family.

It may be reassuring to know that most young people do try drugs at some stage but very few go on to develop a damaging drug habit. Also, drug taking *in itself* is not a risk for HIV but it can involve other risks. The main one is sharing equipment ('works') used for injecting. The risk of HIV can be reduced in the following ways:

Use other ways of taking drugs Sniffing, smoking and eating drugs do not involve risk of HIV.

Don't share works It is very risky for users to share their works with someone else even if they are a good friend, lover or family. A sterile needle and syringe should be used each time. Needle exchange schemes (available in most areas – ring the National Drugs Helpline for details) can supply new works, safely dispose of used works, and provide information on HIV and AIDS.

If absolutely necessary to share works, clean them Drug-using equipment can be cleaned with bleach and clean water, but this is very much a last resort. Full information on this is available from drugs dependency units or specialist HIV agencies (again, via the National Drugs Helpline).

Another risk associated with both drug use and drinking is that people lose their sense of judgement when 'under the influence': many drug users have contracted HIV not through injecting drugs but through unsafe sex.

Transmission through work or social contact

The risk of contracting HIV through social or workplace contact is nearly nil. HIV is a relatively fragile virus: so fragile that even in the most 'risky' workplaces – hospitals – there have been very few cases of workplace transmission. The cases we know about mainly involve needlestick injuries, when a healthworker has accidentally stabbed themselves with a needle contaminated with infected blood. Even in these accidents – when infected blood has gone straight into the bloodstream – few have gone on to become HIV positive. So there should be little cause for concern.

There are, of course, other far more contagious infections that *can* be passed on through casual contact. Simple health and safety precautions will guard against these: for example, cuts and skin wounds covered with waterproof dressings, cleaning up blood and body fluid spillages with diluted bleach, and avoiding direct contact with body fluids where possible. Following these basic hygiene precautions will dramatically cut the risk of any kind of infection – let alone HIV.

These rules may seem like a lot to remember, but it's quite easy if people just make sure that blood, semen or vaginal fluids from someone else don't get into their bloodstream. Until scientists have found a vaccine or a cure, prevention is still the most effective defence against HIV and AIDS.

3.
When someone close has *HIV or AIDS*

Betty's story

Betty is 66 years old. Three and a half years ago her son, Michael, died with AIDS. For the last eighteen months of his life, Michael – an actor in his mid-30s – lived with Betty who cared for him round the clock.

" *You have no idea of the difficulties involved. It's very, very tiring being a carer at this age. All the lifting and carrying – and Michael was so heavy. Like many people my age, I had moved from the family home into a small flat, and suddenly it was crowded out with Michael and his possessions. I felt that I had no space to call my own.*

I also had to cope with Michael's friends. Even though I thought I was open minded, in the beginning I had great problems with these gay friends sitting around telling gay jokes – some of which were very explicit. So this was a whole new culture that I knew nothing about, and I think it took me time to get over it.

But it's not just the caring, it's all of a sudden being 'Mummy' again. It's very tiring, because you have no more life of your own. You submerge your own identity totally, which as you get older is very difficult because you become more set in your ways. You are Mummy and you have no identity. You want to be there and you want to do all this caring bit, but you also want to be able to shut off for a little while, and say, 'I'm going to see a friend of mine, and talk about you and my problems with you', and you can't do that. **"**

Since Michael's death Betty has become very active as an AIDS campaigner. She feels she has had some hostile reaction to her refusal to behave 'like a grandmother'.

  ❝ *I think people see me as a bit of a freak. I have various labels – the grieving mother, the Jewish big mouth, the campaigner and the charity worker. But people also think, 'who the hell does she think she is, at her age?'*

Older people get ignored because of the ageist society we live in. But older people are productive – they can do things that they've never had time for before. And they're not deaf, you don't have to shout at them, and yet they're treated like children – you don't give them credit for being thinking, normal adults.

Older people have a great befriending role: they have something in common with AIDS patients as they're also facing imminent death. Young people feel embarrassed talking about death just as older people feel embarrassed talking about sex – we can help each other! **❞**

Betty also feels that older people may have special needs concerning HIV, particularly after bereavement.

  ❝ *Grandparents feel that they were going to be buried by the grandchild, and they end up burying their own children and grandchildren. They feel cheated, and do not understand how nature has turned the whole thing upside down.* **❞**

Over 20,000 people are known to be infected with HIV in England and Wales alone. Most of them will have family and friends who also feel its impact upon their lives, and many of these are older people. Some of them are the parents of people with HIV, others are grandparents. They may be the husbands, wives or partners of people with HIV infection; or sisters, brothers or other relatives. The connection need not be a blood tie: they may be friends or neighbours or work colleagues. They may be living fairly distant from the person with HIV – perhaps isolated or even estranged. Or they may be providing intensive care and support. It is not known exactly how many older people are in these kinds of situations, but it would not be unreasonable to suggest that the full total could be many thousands.

Of course, all diseases affect other people as well as the individual with the diagnosis. And it is certainly not the intention of this book to suggest that HIV and AIDS should be given some kind of special status as the most uniquely horrible fate that can befall anybody. But many families faced with a diagnosis of HIV do have to deal with some particularly difficult issues.

The first of these is that, for many people, telling their loved ones they are HIV positive also involves disclosure of how they got the virus – and this may mean bringing out into the open some aspect of their behaviour or lifestyle that others may find difficult to acknowledge or accept. Many families find it very hard to deal with open 'proof' that one of their number has been using drugs, or having homosexual sex, or indeed having any sex at all.

Even the most unprejudiced and accepting of families, however, may fear the undoubted stigma still surrounding HIV and AIDS. Everyone has heard horror stories about people with HIV or AIDS (or thought to be at risk) losing their jobs, losing their homes, being banned from public facilities and even physically assaulted. There is still a widespread attitude that AIDS is a self-inflicted disease, and people with HIV are sometimes subject to verbal and physical harassment at the hands of others. The families and friends of people with HIV know and fear this prejudice.

People also find a diagnosis of HIV hard to handle because of the unpredictability of the disease. The progress of HIV through to AIDS and finally death may take months or many years; people may get very ill, then recover and be well again for long periods; many different illnesses may affect someone during the course of HIV, and there is no telling what illness will finally prove fatal or when it will come. Those close to the person with HIV often feel as though they are living on an emotional rollercoaster, in which they keep dropping everything to cope with a severe illness – and maybe prepare themselves for imminent death – only to find that the person recovers and everything has to get 'back to normal' – at least until the next time. Over a period of years, people may go through multiple episodes of fear, exhaustion, grieving and bereavement. This is extremely stressful, and may leave people exhausted and guiltily wondering when the end will finally come.

Telling and hearing

When someone has been diagnosed with HIV, they face difficult choices about whom to tell and when. Within a family situation, these choices may be complicated by past conflicts, or present secrets, relating to sexuality or drug use. Research has found that people with HIV are highly selective about to whom they disclose their HIV status. Many dread causing severe distress to their parents, and choose not to tell parents or brothers and sisters until severe or terminal illness makes it absolutely necessary.

Perhaps even more difficult than causing distress to parents, however, is causing distress to children. Parents may worry that telling their children they have HIV may also involve telling them how they got it, and that their children will be shocked or disgusted or rejecting. Parents feel responsible for their children; they want to protect them and always be there for them. They may feel guilt – particularly if they contracted HIV through sex – that they put their own needs before parental duty and are now having to let down their children. Or they may simply fear that their children will feel abandoned or betrayed.

If the person with HIV has taken the family into their confidence from the beginning, there may be several years before they become ill. This gives the family valuable time in which to come to terms with the situation and understand what the future may bring. But for many families this knowledge comes abruptly and often causes a panicked, thoughtless response.

When people are frightened, they find it hard to think or talk calmly about the implications of the situation facing them. Faced with the disclosure of a loved one's HIV status, many people react with shock, denial and anger. Sometimes there is also fear, guilt and shame, and rejection is not uncommon – one American study found that over one-third of its HIV-positive respondents had been turned away by their families after disclosure.

In their turn, families must then decide whom they are going to tell about the situation they are in. There is evidence that older people find this particularly difficult, and often feel unable to tell anyone at all. The stigma and prejudice surrounding HIV and AIDS – the taboo, the fear of contamination, the moral judgements – are still very powerful disincentives to disclosure. And older people, so often living in communities that may be unsympathetic, with small and shrinking networks of friends, may feel especially silenced.

Sometimes they are frightened that, if they tell anyone, resulting gossip will make life even harder for their loved ones. Doreen Langbridge's son Philip died with AIDS. Her experience, living in a small village, was that neighbours, caring professionals and even some of her friends and family didn't want to know. She found this very painful, and felt forced to retreat into a certain amount of privacy:

“ *We could only tell certain people because we didn't want Philip hurting any more than he was already hurting. We didn't want people shunning him, shutting the door in his face.* ”

Even within families, there is often secrecy and silence about HIV and AIDS. It is not unknown for someone to be seriously ill with HIV disease while actually living with their family, some of whom know the true situation and some of whom do not. Some interesting family games get played regarding who gets told and who doesn't: often it is the older members of the family who are 'protected' from knowledge – as in 'Don't tell your grandmother, it'll kill her'. Grandparents are often put in the position of carrying an entire family's projected frailties and concerns, even if they are actually perfectly able to cope with the real story.

It is almost impossible to overestimate the pain suffered by older people who cannot share their grief and fears with their friends, spiritual leaders, professional helpers, or even with other family members. In extreme cases, they may become virtual prisoners of prejudice. In the Age Concern London report *A Crisis of Silence: HIV, AIDS and Older People*, the case was reported of an older couple whose son died with AIDS. Terrified that the neighbours might ask after their son – and so possibly find out what had happened – they shut themselves away in their home during daylight hours, emerging only in the evening to buy their groceries at a late night store.

Silencing may be a particular problem for older people who – like Doreen – live in small communities, a long way from specialist counselling and other resources. Similarly, people from ethnic or cultural minority communities will often feel very isolated. They may feel unable to be open about their situation within their own communities, for fear of losing the community support that is so vital when living in a foreign culture. Equally, they often find the specialist agencies alien and irrelevant places, geared as they are to the needs of the cultural majority.

So how does anyone know whom to tell, and when? Specialist counselling is available to help people make these decisions, but it is also worth their thinking through the following questions:

- Who do you feel has a right to know?
- Whom do you trust to keep your confidences?
- Who is in a position to provide practical and emotional support to you?
- Who will listen to you, without making judgements?
- Whom do you love and want to feel close to at this time?

It must be remembered that the person with HIV or AIDS is already coping with enormous pressures: it isn't fair or helpful to blame them for bringing it on the family, neither should they be expected to 'make it up to' the family in some way. Each individual has to find their own way of making peace with the past, and choosing how to live the future.

Issues for parents

It is always a tremendous shock for parents to be told that their child is facing a life-threatening medical condition. It is assumed that parents will die before their children, and so it is very hard to accept when this natural order is overturned. Older parents may feel cheated, as though all their years' investment of love and hard work into raising their child has been thrown back in their face by an unjust world. They may also fear for the future, and wonder who will look after them in their last years – particularly if this is an only child.

Many parents suffer strong feelings of guilt. It is quite natural – though not very helpful – for parents to blame themselves when something awful happens to their children. They may wonder what they could have done differently to prevent it, or feel that they must have done something dreadful to deserve such a punishment.

One common reaction to this guilt is to cast around for others to blame – perhaps the person with HIV or their partner, or the other parent. Another common reaction is to become over-protective, trying to wrap the person with HIV in cotton wool, to protect them from the outside world, to treat them as a young child again.

A major problem for many parents is coming to terms with the source of HIV infection, particularly if this is associated with a lifestyle they find hard to accept – most obviously, homosexuality or drug use.

Prejudice against lesbians and gay men is still widespread in our society. Not all older people share this prejudice, by any means, but a significant number do. Part of this is tied up with fear of what the neighbours might say, part is due to regret at the assumed loss of grandchildren, and part is reaction to the stereotype of gay men as sexually promiscuous and unsafe around small children. To be fair, even well-meaning parents with liberal attitudes find it hard to watch their children grow into sexually active adults, and fear for their future if they deviate from the norms and values they were brought up with. Nevertheless, it is very sad that in the 1990s so many young people are still being rejected by their families on the basis of their sexual orientation.

Drug use is a very difficult problem for families. Many parents, on finding out that a child has been taking drugs, panic and over-react. This is not surprising, as drug education campaigns have tended to imply a short and one-way road between drug experimentation and death. Their children, however, have tried drugs and know that one smoke of cannabis – or injection of heroin, come to that – does not make someone a junkie. They know that most drug users do not become addicted and do not die. This gap between their own experience and the views of their parents can lead them to write off the older generation as ignorant fools – and avoid facing up to the very real problems associated with drug use. Although most drug users do not die, many do get into physical, financial, emotional or legal trouble. One of the hardest things for parents to cope with here is their lack of control. Nobody can 'cure' a drug problem except the person with the problem, and drug users really do have to decide for themselves to give up drugs before they can be helped to do so.

Many older parents are also grandparents, and grandparents too face some difficult issues. An unhappy situation that can occur is when grandparents feel they should 'rescue' their grandchildren from living with a parent with HIV. More commonly, however, grandparents stand by their children and find themselves providing practical and emotional support to two generations. Indeed, increasing numbers of older people are caring for grandchildren who have been orphaned through AIDS. Many grandparents feel over-awed at the scale of this task, and the prospect of having to handle many situations that are very new to them (What if the grandchildren are themselves HIV positive? What if they get teased in the playground? What if they have been taken into care?).

It is important for parents and grandparents to talk these issues through carefully and in advance. Unfortunately, many people find it just too painful to talk about the possibility of death, and will put off facing up to these questions for as long as possible. Help is available: St Mary's Hospital in London, for example, runs a group for older carers, and local Age Concern groups may also offer support (see Useful Addresses).

Issues for partners, husbands and wives

Perhaps the relationship that is most vulnerable to a disclosure of HIV is that between partners. 'Partners' is a modern term that many people dislike, but it is used here for want of a better word that includes husbands, wives and unmarried couples whether gay or heterosexual.

For an older person in a long-term relationship, being told that a partner has HIV may shatter the stability and certainties of many years. In some cases, HIV may have been contracted through extra-marital sex, and the partner will be facing the pain of betrayal as well as fears about their own possible infection.

Most older people with HIV are men who contracted the virus via sex with other men. Others have become infected through extra-marital heterosexual sex – often while working or holidaying away from home, and sometimes with prostitutes. Whatever these men's sexual identity, it is not uncommon for them to be married. Their wives have to cope with a double shock – the disclosure of the be-trayal (the past loss) and the knowledge of their husband's condition (the future loss). They will also have to consider whether they them-selves are infected. Not surprisingly, these women may experience a strong sense of injustice when AIDS visits their lives.

Eva Heymann, who runs the Terrence Higgins Trust's Family Support Network, explains it this way:

❝ *The loneliness of these women is unique. For example, a woman may have been married for 23 years, and she finds out her husband has the virus. It's like opening a can of worms. Has he been unfaithful all the time? Is he bisexual? And then, do they tell their grown-up children that their father has the virus? Do they tell their grandchildren? To cope with all that at*

their age is very, very difficult. Often these women will say, 'I feel dirty':
they need very sensitive support. 99

For some, the source of transmission may cause trauma and loss of trust; for others, fear of infection may make it impossible to enjoy a relaxed sexual relationship. Feelings of resentment and envy may surface if one partner is positive and the other is not; equally, when both partners are positive the practical and psychological impact of HIV can snowball.

Practical and financial problems also arise. Plans for the future will be thrown into disarray as the couple try to regain a sense of what their future has to offer. An older partner may assume the responsibility of caring, or both partners may end up caring for each other. The poverty, fatigue, lack of privacy and lack of support that are so common among carers can place an unbearable strain on even the closest relationships.

Because older people often have smaller networks of friendship than the young, the loss of a central, long-term relationship can leave them isolated and bereft. Indeed, as people grow older they frequently face multiple bereavements as friends and relatives age and die, and for many older people the loss of their partner may mean that they live out their own lives totally alone. They may also be left poor or even homeless: this can be a particular problem for older gay men, who lack legal rights and who may be ostracised by their partner's family and heirs. Unless they are lucky enough to have their own networks of informal support, older gay men will not find it easy to locate appropriate bereavement care.

Kingsley's story

Kingsley is aged 67, and is a full-time carer. His companion J'Alex – who is a friend rather than a lover – is 31 and has AIDS. J'Alex has been very ill since March 1994, and Kingsley looks after him round the clock. Although he has his own home, Kingsley now spends more and more time at J'Alex's flat as his caring role has developed.

> *When I first knew him he was very fit and well. But he's developed a kind of dependency on me, so now I find it difficult not to be around even when he's feeling better – there's an emotional leaning as well as physical.*

J'Alex has suffered from shingles, thrush, loss of appetite and constant vomiting. Kingsley deals with all the practical details: changing bedclothes, helping him to the toilet, doing the shopping and cleaning. He does not feel that his age is a problem for him as a carer.

> *I've always been an extremely adaptable person, so I can cope with change pretty well – I'm a tough old bird, actually. Of course it's a strain – it would be a strain on anybody – but I am a strong sort of character, and my physical strength has been really good. Sure, there have been times when I've been physically exhausted, but so would anybody, so I wouldn't say I was that different from a younger carer.*

However, caring for J'Alex has changed Kingsley's life dramatically. He finds it hard to keep up old activities – for example, he was Secretary for an Age Concern group – and he finds his social life is now centred around J'Alex's flat.

Practical help is obtained from Crossroads Care, which provides home support services, and from a local HIV drop-in centre. Meals on Wheels are delivered by The Food Chain, which provides cooked meals to people who are homebound because of HIV.

Kingsley feels that in many ways his age can be an advantage:

> *I've taken on a fatherly role. I think older people regard illness and death in a somewhat different light to younger people. Without being morbid, I'd say I was in the last stage of my life cycle, so the idea of death doesn't worry me as much as it might have done when I was younger. The older you are, the more bereavements you have, so I'm probably more used to death and can take it more in my stride. The idea of dying doesn't particularly depress me.*

Generally, he doesn't think that enough has been done to help older people affected by HIV and AIDS:

“People are beginning to wake up to the fact that there are older people around who have lives to lead and need support and are able to give support, and I think it's only in the last few years that this has been addressed.”

He feels that the most important area that needs addressing is education, particularly with regard to sexuality. The problem lies in breaking down the barriers created by older people who are not used to discussing sexual matters.

“People of my generation were brought up in a secret world, and there wasn't the information available. There were very few clubs, and they were mainly underground. We never identified ourselves as being gay people, we were just doing our own thing, quietly and without talking about it, because of the social attitudes and the legal implications as well. So a lot of older people aren't fully integrated as they still have that background of secrecy.

A lot of straight older people affected by HIV and AIDS are probably more secretive than gay people because of the stigma – despite education, it's still considered a gay disease. They were brought up never to talk about sexuality anyway, and the subject of HIV and AIDS is highly emotive, so they would tend to be more secretive and less forthcoming, and the more secretive you are, the less well informed you become.”

Kingsley is also Chair of the Libertines, a support group for older gay men attached to Age Concern. The group meets fortnightly, and has an average attendance of between 12 and 20 people. Although Kingsley has tried to encourage discussion of HIV issues in the group, he has not found this easy.

“Older gay people don't want to talk about it so much and older straight people probably don't want to talk about it at all. Some of them are very ill informed. One of them said to me once, 'I see my doctor regularly, so if I had AIDS he would tell me.' So there's certainly a need for education, but they don't really want to talk about gay matters, and certainly not in a serious way. A number of our members are married, and the whole of their life is clouded in secrecy. The others, too, have learned to be secretive over the years.

It's difficult for them to join the group anyway. We see people walking up and down outside, trying to pluck up the courage to come in. We have quite a number of people who don't want to think in gay terms at all. They enjoy mixing and relaxing and not having to watch their tongues – as they have to in straight company – but they don't want to talk about anything serious.

Also, because they're older, they don't want to talk about death as they know that they're nearer to it than younger people. Even if they had a pamphlet shoved in front of their face they might not read it – they just don't want to know about it. 99

One of the ways in which Kingsley has tried to confront this problem was to bring together the Libertines, Age Concern and The Positive Place (an HIV centre) to produce leaflets on HIV and AIDS and safer sex specifically for older people. They have published a leaflet for older heterosexuals, and one for older gay men: in each case, they tried to use language that older people can relate to. These leaflets – and accompanying posters – have proved extremely popular.

HIV, AIDS and relationships

The challenge of AIDS can destroy relationships – and also rebuild them. Many people find that they lose friends who cannot cope with them having HIV, but that for those who remain the friendships are strengthened and deepened. There really is no blueprint for how HIV and AIDS could affect someone's family. Everyone likes to think that suffering can bring them together and make them better people – like poor little Beth in *Little Women*, oozing goodness from her deathbed. The reality is that pain does not make people pure, and if a person has always had a difficult relationship with someone they will probably find that their HIV diagnosis won't transform it. Even if a person has had a close relationship, it can sometimes be hard to handle anger, blame, guilt, exhaustion and the myriad other feelings that can surface when someone close is terminally ill.

An HIV diagnosis can also put things in their proper perspective, however. People tend to take each other for granted in relationships, and sometimes it is good to be reminded about what the important things in life are really about. Parents may have been angry with their son for years because he turned out to be gay. OK, he's not the son they wanted, but he's the son they've got and this can be seen as a challenge to rebuild the relationship while they can.

If someone has had a difficult relationship, this could be a time for healing and reconciliation. But this should be taken slowly and respectfully. It's easy to get carried away with a prodigal son-type drama, particularly if this is viewed as a kind of deathbed reunion. But it probably won't be a deathbed reunion: people with HIV can and usually do live for many years after diagnosis. It isn't possible to live a relationship as though it's in its last moments. The challenge is to construct a real, whole relationship. Professional help may be needed with this – sources of advice and support are given in the Useful Addresses section.

Living with someone with HIV is not always easy, and it will be necessary for people to make choices about how much of their own life they are prepared to sacrifice to care for a loved one. It is easy to make grand gestures out of genuine compassion – inviting an estranged relative to come and live in their home is one example. But the 'host' needs to make sure that these plans can last the distance, and that other loved ones – their partner, or other children, for example – are not forced into a position of having to make unwilling sacrifices. At the end of the day, everyone is still an individual with the right to live their own life, and HIV and AIDS should not take that away.

4.
HIV and AIDS in later life

Joe's story

Joe is a 70-year-old Anglican clergyman, who is largely retired but still preaches about once a month. For many years Joe worked with the ex-patriate community in Buenos Aires, Argentina. He returned to England after being diagnosed with HIV nine years ago – though he thinks he contracted the virus some 18 months before that. The diagnosis came as a complete shock to him.

66 *I was knocked sideways – struck dumb; and then I just went numb. I really didn't know what to think or what to do. I think this is a fairly common experience, and you think you're going to die straight away. In those days, they said only about 10 per cent of people with the virus would develop AIDS, so I thought I'd maybe be one of the 90 per cent who wouldn't . . . but then the news got worse, until they said everybody with HIV would develop AIDS.* 99

Joe decided to move back to England, but at first he found it hard to tell anybody about his condition.

66 *The worst thing was that I didn't dare tell anybody. The publicity about AIDS was horrific, and everybody was terrified of it. Although I had some very good friends, I daren't tell them as I simply didn't know how people were going to react. I thought I might end up without any friends.* 99

Having told his friends and his Church, however, Joe has experienced no prejudice.

❝ *I now make no secret of it at all, and I've had no hostile reaction from anybody ever. The blessing has been that HIV has forced me to come out – in all sorts of ways. It's a truth that makes you free. And now I feel freer than I have ever felt in my life, because I'm not having to hide anything or pretend to be anything I'm not.* **❞**

As Joe's story shows, HIV and AIDS can affect people from every walk of life. The assumption that older people are not at risk from HIV is largely due to the widespread belief that older people do not get up to anything which could possibly put them at risk. Even the medical profession signs up to this prejudice: a survey of doctors and nurses working with older people in Birmingham found that fully 50 per cent did not believe their patients could be at risk from HIV and AIDS.

If geriatricians and other health professionals are not aware that HIV may affect older people, they are not likely to look for it or test it as a possible diagnosis. This suggests that the number of older people with HIV infection may have been under-estimated, and that they may make up a larger proportion of people with AIDS than the current reported total of 11 per cent.

There are other reasons for suggesting that this may be the case. One is that older people with HIV seem to fall sick and die much more quickly than their younger counterparts (although Joe is an example of how this need not be so); another is the increased likelihood that they will die of conditions unrelated to HIV during the 'latent' or symptomless period. HIV illness may present a different clinical picture in older people than among the young: most doctors' knowledge of HIV comes from research on young men, and mounting evidence suggests that other groups – particularly older people and women – may develop different, and perhaps overlooked, symptoms.

Finally, symptoms of HIV illness in older people often resemble other, age-related diseases and so may escape detection. For example, the first symptom of AIDS in older people is often dementia. Whilst dementia in young people is rare and demands immediate investigation, in older people it is likely to be mistaken for Alzheimer's-related ('senile') dementia and treated as such. Yet as people with HIV increasingly live for many years after diagnosis, larger numbers of them will survive to reach old age, and so the proportion of older people who are HIV positive will grow.

It is not just doctors who are unaware of HIV and AIDS in the elderly, however. Older people themselves, not surprisingly, have by and large accepted the 'common sense' view that they are not affected, even though many of them have been or continue to be at risk. Older people are recipients of more blood products and organ transplants than any other age group, and before 1985 this was a major source of HIV infection (donated blood is now screened, and blood products are heat-treated to kill the virus).

Even older people who are sexually active do not necessarily see HIV and AIDS as an issue for them. In one American study of older people, 51 per cent of the women and 92 per cent of the men said they were sexually active. Of these, 12 per cent had received blood transfusions between 1977 and 1985 but *none* used condoms or had been tested for HIV.

There is very little information on HIV and AIDS aimed at older people. To be sure, there is no shortage of leaflets, posters and advertisements telling people about HIV, AIDS and safer sex, but they are targeted at a younger audience. In order to be attractive and effective for young people, they use streetwise language, modern slang, trendy design and images of young people. Unfortunately, this means they don't work well for older audiences – in fact, older people are more likely to think these materials are not meant for them and have nothing to say to them.

The other places where young people learn about HIV and AIDS – sex education classes, family planning clinics, youth media – are similarly out of bounds for elderly people. Of course targeting information at younger people is vital, but it must be remembered that older people also have difficulty in asking and talking about sex. And so do the professionals who work with them. Teachers and youth club leaders will usually have far more training and know-how to help them respond to questions about sex and sexuality than will geriatric nurses or residential care staff.

Virtually the only leaflets on HIV and AIDS that have older people specifically in mind come from Age Concern organisations that produce leaflets for older gay men and for older people generally: details are given in the Further Reading section.

Although there are signs that awareness of this issue is growing, it is undoubtedly true that, for the first decade of AIDS in the United Kingdom, older people as a whole were badly let down, neglected by HIV educators and overlooked by health workers.

How older people are at risk from HIV

Blood products

In the years 1979–1985, before blood donations were routinely screened and Factor VIII treatment for haemophilia was heat-treated, these were routes for HIV transmission. Around the world, this has been the most common cause of HIV infection among older people, probably because older people are major users of blood products. In the USA, for example, nearly half of all blood transfusions are given to people aged over 60.

The situation is rather different in the United Kingdom, where sexual activity – not blood products – has been the major route of HIV transmission. But we do know of at least 80 cases of HIV in older people due to infected blood products; there may, of course, be more that we don't know about. If someone has had a blood transfusion in the past and is worried that they may have contracted HIV, they can be reassured that the chances of this happening are something like one in a million.

A report in the US journal *Geriatrics* tells the case of a 90-year-old man, Mr A, a German immigrant who settled in the USA in 1936. In 1983, Mr A had a stomach operation requiring transfusion of several pints of blood. In 1987, while travelling in Austria, Mr A went into a local hospital with an acute diarrhoeal illness. It is routine Austrian policy that all foreigners who attend a hospital undergo HIV testing. Mr A was tested and found to have HIV infection.

By November 1988, Mr A had developed dementia and pneumonia. His decline was rapid thereafter, and he died from pneumonia in January 1989. The authors of the report recommend that HIV should always be considered when older people go to their doctor with a history of transfusion and symptoms of pneumonia or dementia.

Men who have sex with men

If popular prejudice likes to pretend that older people don't have sex, then older people who have homosexual sex are practically invisible. It seems to be easier to believe that homosexuals are all young men in tight jeans who were born after 1967 (when sex between men was partially decriminalised). It is not known how many older people are homosexual: one study estimates there are around 400,000 homosexual men aged over 60 in England and Wales, while others suggest a formula of one in ten. The most comprehensive research of recent years, the National Sex Survey, didn't include anybody over pensionable age, unfortunately. But any such estimates must be treated with caution, because sexual identity is not fixed and may vary over time or in different circumstances.

Most of us talk about sexual orientation as fixed and self-evident: we assume that the categories 'homosexual' and 'heterosexual' are discrete and unchanging; that everyone 'knows' their sexual identity and sticks to it; that you cannot love one person and sleep with another; that we can tell if someone close to us is gay. None of these assumptions bears much resemblance to the reality of people's lived experience, and none of them is helpful to an understanding of the spread of HIV and AIDS.

Among older age groups, homosexual behaviour is more likely to be kept secret. It is also less likely to be tied to a homosexual identity: large numbers of older gay men are bisexual and many are married, combining a heterosexual identity with homosexual behaviour. This is not unique to older men: opportunistic sexual activity occurs in all-male institutions among heterosexual men; bisexuality is common and both 'straight' and 'gay' men often experiment sexually.

Older men often find it more difficult to be open about their sexuality: they will have grown up in the pre-1967 days, when homosexual practices were illegal, and this may still influence their sexual identity and behaviour. They are less likely to be 'out' on the gay scene (and its networks of HIV-related information and support): some may rely on casual sexual encounters, whilst others find it difficult to meet enough prospective sexual partners to build up the experience and confidence to practise safer sex. It can be especially difficult for married men who engage in illicit, unsafe sex to go home and start practising safer sex – for example by suggesting condom use to a wife who is past the menopause or is using another form of contraception.

A number of older gay men interviewed anonymously for this book complained that they have never seen information on HIV, AIDS and safer sex that addressed their particular needs. They understood and approved of the commitment of AIDS organisations to educating young gay men, particularly those who are 'new on the scene', as many of them are at high risk of contracting and passing on HIV. However, they felt that health promotion materials covered with young models, using slang they didn't understand and distributed through nightclubs and other 'youth' venues, couldn't work for them. Almost by definition, a successfully targeted health promotion campaign must leave others uneducated – and that is exactly what has happened to older men.

Elizabeth's story

Elizabeth is 58 years old and Ugandan; she has lived in England for seven years. She used to be a hairdresser/beautician, but no longer works. She was married, but has been divorced for 12 years. She has five children: the eldest is 34, the youngest 25.

Elizabeth was diagnosed HIV positive in 1989, and is now showing symptoms of AIDS. She believes she contracted the virus sexually from a boyfriend.

66 *I went for a blood transfusion and had a plaster on my arm. When he saw the plaster he never came back again – he just disappeared. I suspected then that he had given me the virus. I didn't trust him much. I think he may have slept with men as well as women.* 99

Since her diagnosis, Elizabeth has suffered from chest problems, diarrhoea and depression. She kept her diagnosis secret for nearly three years, eventually told one of her daughters, and has recently told the rest of her children.

66 *I kept it to myself for quite a long time. I used to go to this clinic every two weeks, and they told me to go to one of these support groups but I refused. I was feeling so bad I just wanted to die. Now I go to Body Positive, and it helps me. I think if I hadn't had this I would have been dead long ago – or in a mental hospital – because I couldn't bear it, I didn't know what to do with myself. But the people here are my friends now: I call them my sisters.* 99

She has two or three friends outside the group but will never tell them.

66 *You never know how people are going to react. I'd be rejected by most people; they would fear me. They have to be educated, and until they are it has to be like this.* 99

Elizabeth, like many people, assumed she was not at risk from HIV because she was not gay:

66 *I don't know how I thought I couldn't get it. I thought it was only gay men who could get the illness, and that's where I went wrong. I never thought it could spread to heterosexuals* 99

and because she was not young:

66 *If you're an older woman, and you're divorced and have got older kids, people don't expect you to have a boyfriend. And I've got grandchildren as well. They expect you to just sit in the house and sleep. But I still needed to enjoy myself, just like anybody else. Perhaps I would have been more careful before my menopause as I wouldn't have wanted to have another baby. But I could no longer have children, and I could have been free – if it wasn't for this virus.* 99

Elizabeth sees both advantages and disadvantages to facing the challenge of AIDS at her age.

66 *It doesn't matter whether you're old or young: the virus doesn't select an age, and you're facing the same thing. But I suppose I feel I'm lucky because I've got my children. If I'd had the virus before, I would have been too scared to have kids – to bring up a baby and then leave it behind when I died. Younger women who haven't had children haven't been able to enjoy their lives.*

I'm very proud of my age, and I don't fear death. But I do fear that I'll be weaker because I'm older, and that people will be less sympathetic. They might think that, because I'm older, I should have known what I was doing.

When I'm feeling very sick I don't even want to be in London. I wish I could just go off in isolation and die there. I don't want people to know, as they might reject my children. Maybe they would be supportive, but how do I know that? That's my general feeling: I just want to protect myself and my children. People fear this virus. 99

Transmission between men and women

Older people are not immune from heterosexual transmission of HIV: unfortunately, neither are they immune from the widespread complacency that AIDS is not an issue for those with 'normal' lifestyles.

Not all older people are married or in long-term relationships. Those who are may not be sexually faithful. A significant proportion of older people will have started new relationships within the past decade: these include the widowed and the divorced, as well as the never-married. Older people in search of new sexual partners after bereavement or the end of a long-term relationship may be more ignorant of the risks of HIV than many young people. They will not have had recent sex education, or attended a family planning clinic, or watched a government advertisement directed at them. Although it is important to keep the level of risk in perspective, it is easy for older people to deny altogether their risk of contracting HIV.

Both married women and men may engage in secret adulterous affairs. And both heterosexual and homosexual older men may use prostitutes – again without their partner's knowledge. Whilst prostitutes, generally speaking, have good knowledge of safer sex, they are sometimes bribed or pressured by clients into not using a condom.

Older people in all these situations have two things in common. The first is that although they, like most heterosexuals, may continue to believe that they are not at risk, many of them cannot be sure that this is also true for their sexual partners. The second is that most older people will have grown up in a time and culture that discouraged open discussion of sexuality and sexual health. Although this is not to suggest that all older people find it hard to express their feelings, it is certainly true that many will have had a lifetime's training in denying their own sexual needs (particularly women) and emotional needs (particularly men). Most of us find it difficult to discuss and negotiate safer sex: for people who have been silenced by years of taboos and prejudice, it can be very, very hard to develop the confidence, self-knowledge and vocabulary to do this effectively.

Reg's story

Reg is 60 years old, and a retired decorator. Four years ago he was diagnosed HIV positive, and last year he developed AIDS. Reg says he has no idea how he contracted AIDS, but assumes it was through sex. His diagnosis was not altogether a surprise, and he has always been open about it.

66 *The biggest problem is the secrecy. I have a pet theory that more people die from fright than from the disease. The word kills them. Once you've accepted that it is a complaint, you've accepted 50 per cent of the battle. If you are made afraid of it, then you're in terrible trouble because you're not going to know how to react or fight. If the fight is taken away from you, you have nothing.* 99

Reg is very aware that HIV symptoms may get confused with, or exaggerate, the normal ageing process.

66 *Getting flu when you're older can be much worse than when you're younger, and HIV is much the same. AIDS does seem rather different with an old person, but the medical profession often don't understand that. You have to make sure you're seeing someone who understands that, just because you're a certain age, senility is not something that's coming along because of old age – it's because of HIV infection.*

AIDS exaggerates your physical disabilities. You're not as able to do a lot of things – even walking sometimes. It also affects my brain. As you get older you get more forgetful, but for me the forgetfulness is coming on earlier. For example, the other day I fancied making a sandwich, so I went to get a plate to put it on and found I didn't have any. It worried me, so I went to lie down in bed, and I heard a clank. I turned the top cover down and found I had put the plates in bed. These are the kinds of things that happen.

I've always said that I could survive without my arms and legs so long as I have a brain. But that's a joke where I'm concerned because the first thing that will go wrong with me is my brain, and that's the most active thing I've used and the thing I find hardest to shut off. I can't have conversations in groups for more than two hours: I start to feel like an idiot and probably sound like one as well. 〞

Reg is critical of the doctors he has faced.

〝 *They don't have much experience of handling people of an older age. They were slightly patronising – they treated me in the same way as if I had just come out of hospital and needed to recuperate.*

The medical profession hasn't geared itself to older people. They still think of it as a young person's disease. There's very little information about people over 50. Once they become ill, they go into the category of pensioners and geriatrics. When they're diagnosing an older person, the medical profession must be aware that what they could be diagnosing is an HIV infection, as well as something that could be part of a normal age deterioration. They've got to look out for both now, and not assume someone is too old for HIV. 〞

Reg thinks that older people are often reluctant to talk openly about sexual issues, and that this causes problems for them in coming to terms with HIV and AIDS.

〝 *There's such stigma. Older people are afraid of talking about sex, and of talking about feelings. Sometimes they can't get through the taboo: one old dear I met said, 'It's the plague; it's retribution for homosexuals'. When I pointed out that anybody could get it, even children, she said, 'I don't believe it'.*

And older homosexuals are also reluctant to be open. An older homosexual guy would have been closeted for years and years because he was brought up in that period when you couldn't come out because of family, work and social status in the community – but he may 'let himself go' on holiday [have an affair with another man]. He knows the helping organisations are there, but he can't go because he thinks people will see him as a dirty old man. 〞

He also feels that AIDS organisations are targeting the young and ignoring older people, and that the information available is not relevant for the elderly.

" *All the stuff being written now is useless. It's street talk or medical jargon. The younger ones can understand it, but the older ones can't. Also, there's information for every other category – unmarried mothers, 18-year-olds, black people – but nothing for older people. AIDS organisations should not only be centred around gay people – they should be helping all of us in one big pot.* "

Reg himself helps other older people affected by HIV or AIDS through his involvement with ACE 50+ (Age Concern and Education for those aged 50 and over). This is a small group, affiliated to the local Age Concern (Hammersmith & Fulham), which acts as a contact and education resource for those interested in HIV and older people.

Reg's own secret for coping with AIDS is:

" *Accepting – it's the key to everything. By accepting it you discover yourself, and change your lifestyle. You can be more healthy. You keep a good diet, don't burn the candle at both ends, relax and enjoy life. Don't think, 'Should I?' Think, 'I will'.* "

Older people's experience of HIV infection

The physical impact

Generally speaking, older people with HIV will have a shorter life expectancy than younger people with HIV. Obviously this statement is about averages: Joe, whose story was told at the beginning of this chapter, is remarkably fit and healthy for anyone of his age, HIV positive or not. There is a shortage of research in this area, but the studies that are available suggest that older people develop HIV illness, and go on to die, more quickly than the young. This is because the ageing process naturally reduces the efficiency of the immune system, thus making older people with HIV more vulnerable to opportunistic infections and cancers.

The first signs of HIV illness in older people are easily confused with other diseases suffered by this age group. A French study reports that the major characteristic of AIDS in older people is the high percentage of patients who have major neurological and psychiatric disorders, including encephalitis (brain inflammation). They suggest that many older people with these kinds of conditions may have been wrongly diagnosed as having Alzheimer's disease, which is a medical condition that affects more people, the older they become. Similarly, PCP (the type of pneumonia that is common among people with AIDS) has been mistaken for lung disease and heart failure.

HIV disease tends to be more aggressive among older people. One reason for this is the severity of the encephalitis; another is that initial misdiagnosis – which we suspect is common among older people with HIV – will mean late recognition and delayed treatment. It is important to remember, however, that older people are also benefiting from the rapid developments in delaying the onset of AIDS and in treating HIV-related disease.

Healthcare is not unlimited, and older people may be among the most likely losers. Resources are – generally speaking – weighted in favour of the young. It is important, then, for older people to keep informed about their own health and to assert their own claims for treatment. Everyone finds this difficult, unfortunately, and it may be that older people – brought up at a time when doctors were authority figures – may find this especially hard.

A problem that worsens the prognosis for older people with HIV is the poverty that affects all too many older people in the United Kingdom. The commonest health advice to people with HIV illness is to eat a balanced, high-protein diet, to keep warm and comfortable and to avoid stress. In 1991, a joint study by the Bloomsbury & Islington Health Authority and the Terrence Higgins Trust found that the average cost of a high-protein diet in London was £42 per week. People living on low incomes cannot afford this. Furthermore, older people often live in poor quality housing that is difficult and costly to keep warm and dry.

People aged 65 or over are not eligible for certain important benefits, such as Invalid Care Allowance and cash payments from the Independent Living Fund. But perhaps the most damaging loss is their ineligibility to claim Disability Living Allowance (DLA), which is non-means-tested, non-taxable, can be paid on top of other benefits without reducing their value, and is the key to a number of other benefits and services. Attendance Allowance is an alternative to DLA but it does not include a 'mobility component' for people who need help getting about. The Terrence Higgins Trust states:

66 *It is difficult to exaggerate the importance of DLA to people living with symptomatic [active] HIV or AIDS. Getting this benefit can lead to significant increases in income which could make an enormous difference to their quality of life.* 99

Further information and advice on this can be found in Chapter 6.

The emotional impact

Someone who has been diagnosed with HIV will, of course, experience emotional and psychological reactions common to anyone with an HIV diagnosis – or, indeed, any life-threatening illness. These include denial, anger, depression and guilt. But older people are particularly likely to suffer these emotions in isolation. Compared to young people, they may not have a wide network of friends, and many of their long-standing friends may already be dead.

If they are gay, they may be estranged from their family of origin. Or they may be living with their family but unable to be open about their sexual orientation or their HIV status. Or they may live on their own. Whatever their personal situation, it is not often that an older person with HIV will feel able to discuss their situation openly with neighbours, professional helpers or friends. In one case, a woman in her late 70s reported that her HIV status had caused her less trauma than the reaction from family and professional helpers alike to the knowledge that she was still sexually active.

People with HIV or AIDS have done much to support each other through the development of self-help groups and the provision of user-led services. However, much of this is a product of the young, gay culture from which it came, and is inaccessible and intimidating to older people and particularly to older women. Even older gay men may feel alienated from these services, because so much of gay culture celebrates youth. Whilst it is absolutely right that the majority of people with HIV or AIDS (ie young gay men) should have services that are appropriate to their needs, no one should underestimate the difficulties caused to the minority if they do not have similar access.

This is particularly pertinent where older people are further distanced from mainstream provision by their gender, or ethnic origin, or disability. HIV is not just a medical condition but is also a social phenomenon that highlights deeply held fears and convictions about sexuality, disease and death. These are more than deeply personal issues: they are also culturally specific concerns. Becoming HIV positive may raise special needs and anxieties about isolation, community disapproval and getting appropriate help.

There is much that is not known about the psychological impact of HIV and AIDS on older people, because of their 'invisibility' in the available literature. Some of the people interviewed for this book suggested that the increased shame and isolation suffered by older people could in itself be a partial explanation of their early death after diagnosis. Others, however, feel that older people may have life experience and inner resources that help them to cope rather better with HIV and AIDS than do younger people.

Living with the diagnosis

If someone has been diagnosed with HIV – or is worried that they may be HIV positive – it really does make sense to seek professional help as early as possible. These days people can and do live for years with an HIV diagnosis, and proper medical help can make a real difference to their quality of life.

It's important to get emotional and practical support, too. Joe, Reg and Elizabeth's stories all illustrate the value of people being able to share their situation with others – and of keeping involved and active for as long as possible. There is a full list of support organisations in the Useful Addresses section.

The experience of HIV and AIDS varies for every individual, but, given the right help and support, they can carry on feeling in control of their life. The following chapters discuss ways in which to start getting that help and support.

5.
Living with HIV and AIDS

Planning for the future

Whether someone has HIV infection or is a friend or relative of someone with the virus, they will need to plan for the future. Even if the person with HIV is currently fit, healthy and coping with life, it is likely that the time will come when their needs for medical and social care will become high.

It is important not to be panicked into hasty decisions, however. Someone with an HIV diagnosis may – indeed, is likely – to go on living for many years. Any plans that are made must be sensible and flexible enough to last.

This chapter sets out some of the issues people may have to face when they or someone they care for has HIV or AIDS. Following on from previous chapters, it looks at the progression of HIV disease, and its likely impact on a person's physical and emotional well-being. The organisations listed in the Useful Addresses section aim to offer a wide range of support and services. Chapter 6 goes on to provide advice on some of the practical issues they may face about housing, money, daily living and medical care and – finally – about death and bereavement.

HIV disease: what to expect

There is no model of HIV disease that holds true for everybody: as has already been said, individuals experience the disease in very different ways, and most of the medical conditions associated with HIV can also affect people who do not have the virus. So it is vitally important that someone reading the following does not take it as some kind of blueprint for how HIV will progress. No book is able to give that kind of information. Nevertheless, it may be useful to sketch out a common framework for the progression of HIV disease.

When people are first infected with HIV, they may develop an infection lasting a week or two. For some people, these symptoms are so mild they go unnoticed, whilst others feel more ill as with a nasty bout of flu. At this stage the individual may not have a positive result to an HIV test. It may be several weeks until 'seroconversion' takes place – that is, the body develops antibodies to HIV that can be detected.

There may then be a long period when the person feels well and functions normally – except, perhaps, for the emotional stress of a positive test result. This is called the asymptomatic period, and often lasts for many years.

After a period of time (commonly five to eight years but, again, with considerable individual variation) most people start developing conditions such as thrush, shingles, weight loss, diarrhoea and a host of possible others. As they become more seriously ill, common conditions include Kaposi's sarcoma (tumour of the blood vessels), PCP (a type of pneumonia) and tuberculosis. Women often suffer gynaecological conditions such as pelvic inflammatory disease and cervical cancer, and there is some evidence that older people are particularly prone to developing HIV-related dementia (although this occurs in about 30–50 per cent of all people with late-stage severe AIDS).

Every individual experiences HIV disease differently. Some get terminally ill very quickly; others may experience a whole series of different illnesses; others may get so seriously ill that there seems no hope of survival, then recover and are well again for long periods. Of course, people with HIV may also get ill for other reasons: in other words, even if someone is HIV positive and has cancer, the two are not necessarily connected.

At this time, most medical opinion sees AIDS as eventually fatal. There is continuing controversy about this, however, with others arguing that it need not necessarily be so, and increasing numbers of very long-term survivors.

How is someone with an HIV diagnosis to make sense of this mass of sometimes contradictory information, and with such wide individual variation? Everyone has different ways of dealing with this, but many people with HIV have chosen to become their own best doctors, finding out as much as they can about the condition, and learning to read their own body's signals.

How people feel

Anyone who has been diagnosed with a life-threatening disease will, of course, suffer some kind of emotional reaction. Again, there is no blueprint of how someone will react to this kind of stress, and the psychological resources people bring to any given situation will influence how they respond to it. Older people often have greater inner strength and stamina, built up over a lifetime of dealing with stressful experiences. However, they are also more likely than the young to be lonely and isolated, lacking close relationships with people they would want to confide in.

When they are told of a positive diagnosis with HIV, people may have particular problems with the uncertainty of their situation. Feeling that their world has been knocked off kilter, they may want certainty about what how they will get ill and when, about how other people will react, about what the future will bring. Sadly, these certainties are not available.

The individual variations in how HIV disease progresses, and the long periods during which many people remain perfectly well, cause their own difficulties. For some people – or their loved ones – it can feed denial of the reality of their situation. Others may anxiously monitor every cough or cold for signs of disease. Some may do everything possible to blot out the pain of their situation – perhaps through drink or drugs. Others may dedicate their lives to special diets, health regimens, AIDS activism. What is denial and what is obsession? What is fatalism and what is healthy acceptance? There are no rules, no ideal way for people to behave. Unfortunately, people with HIV – or those close to them – often feel that they *should* be reacting in a certain way, and feel judged accordingly by those around them.

During periods of ill health, people face even more stress. They will have to cope with a whole range of illnesses, medications, medical procedures and perhaps repeated hospitalisation. They may be troubled by their increasing dependency, and by hopelessness in the face of impending death. The following are some common emotional reactions.

Depression

Depression is often under-estimated as just feeling a bit sad. In fact, it can be an extremely difficult and prolonged condition, with symptoms including tiredness, loss of energy, low self-esteem, no interest in the outside world, weepiness, over- or under-eating, complete loss of hope.

Depression may be caused simply by the situation the person is in, but it may also be a result of HIV-related illness or a side effect of medication. It is important that people with HIV don't give up hope: there is always *something* that can be done to improve quality of life. Some people find that depression lifts if they talk it over with someone they trust, give themselves little treats or pursue outside interests. If the problem is more severe, counselling, therapy or medication may help.

Fear

People often fear what they do not understand and cannot control. People with HIV – and those close to them – may be very scared of what the future will bring. They may over-react to normal fluctuations in well-being, seeing every cough and rash as a symptom of AIDS. They may devise nightmare scenarios in their heads, in which everything that could possibly go wrong will go wrong.

Getting informed about HIV and AIDS can help to lessen any fear of the unknown. Many people also find it useful to join self-help groups, to meet others affected by HIV. Counselling and therapy can also be helpful.

Anger

'Why me?' people ask. A diagnosis of HIV seems so unfair – perhaps particularly to parents who have worked hard to raise a child, only to see them face a life-threatening disease. Anger may be directed inwards, resulting in depression, disordered eating, taking drugs or drinking too much. Or it may be directed towards loved ones, or to health professionals and other helping agencies.

People need to be allowed to be angry, and to get it out of their systems. This is tough on the person who is taking the brunt of the anger but they should remember that it is the disease that is the enemy, not themselves. It is important to try to achieve a healthy balance, letting the individual express their anger without getting angry back or shutting them up but not letting them abuse or victimise the person on the 'receiving end'.

Some people successfully redirect their anger by getting involved with AIDS activism, voluntary work or other outside activities.

Guilt

People with HIV may feel guilty for having got the virus, for bringing it into the lives of their loved ones, about the behaviour that put them at risk in the first place. Parents may feel guilty that it happened to their child and not to them, that they should have been able to do something to protect their child. Carers may feel guilty that it is not they that are infected, that they should be able to do more to help.

It is important for everyone to remember that AIDS is not a punishment or a judgement. Understanding *why* they feel guilty may help, perhaps by talking their feelings through with a counsellor or someone they trust.

People have different ways of dealing with these emotional problems. Some become very informed and knowledgeable about HIV, so taking some control over it, while others prefer to ignore it and continue life as normal. Some turn to God, some to support groups. For most, acute distress fades into an understanding that they can live with the virus. A minority become very seriously depressed. Some people change their lives, determined to pursue fulfilment or long-held dreams; others tidy up relationships.

Relationships

Sometimes the person with HIV will put all their energies into coping with the people around them. Parents and carers may be consumed with anxiety. They feel that they should know what the person with HIV feels and wants, and that they should be able to supply it. They may suffer guilt that it's not them who's ill (this is particularly true for mothers). Carers get burnt out – depressed, hostile, impatient, agitated. They think they can't cope, they lose their sense of humour, they have trouble concentrating or sleeping, they over-eat or under-eat or drink or take drugs, they get sick and feel distant from other people.

People with HIV or AIDS sometimes feel unable to reassure their care-givers. They may feel pressure to pretend they're less ill than they are, to minimise the demands on others. Carers often focus on sickness, when the person with HIV wants to focus on other things, to not have to be an object of pity the whole time.

Balancing sympathy and intrusion is difficult. For people dealing with HIV infection, sympathy – both as a blessing and a burden – is as much a fact of life as the infection. At times, people make each other feel comforted and reassured. At other times, people's feelings are so overwhelming that they need to protect themselves from the pain, and just can't help the other person. When this happens, the person with HIV or AIDS and their carer may need a break from each other.

Carers can avoid asking for reassurance that creates a burden or that cannot be given. They can respect the abilities of the person with HIV to find his or her own solutions. They can understand that some things can't be fixed. They can allow the person to talk freely and openly and without interruption or fear of judgement. They can listen, though they find it hard. They can let the person cry, and not try to make them stop. They can allow the person to be alone, and not talk. They can learn to accept their own helplessness in the face of incurable disease.

Particular problems can arise when the person with HIV has parents and a partner – or perhaps an 'alternative family' of close friends. Even previously amicable relationships may become fraught with rivalry over who is the closest to the person with HIV, who has the right to make decisions about their welfare, their funeral, their Will, or interpret their moods and desires.

This is not usually such a problem when the person with HIV is married, because families will usually (though not always) accord some kind of 'rights' to a legal spouse. But where the relationship is less well defined, or is between people of the same sex, families sometimes act as if this person or these people are interlopers into the 'real' relationships of family life. Equally, partners can sometimes resent and resist family involvement – perhaps especially where there is a history of family hostility to this relationship in particular or to homosexuality in general. These are very painful situations, and it is important to try to resolve them without adding stress to the person with HIV by asking them to mediate or to choose.

Dependency and control

No one wants to feel helpless. HIV disease can seriously undermine a person's sense of control and self-worth. Carers may also feel they lack control – over their own lives, or over their ability to put the situation right. Sometimes it can feel as though HIV spreads into the lives of a whole network of people through one individual, ruling all their lives.

It can be difficult to balance comfort and care with independence. At certain times, people with HIV may *want* to be 'babied' – most people find this reassuring at times of illness or vulnerability. At other times, they may feel angry at being patronised. It can be hard for everyone to cope with needs that are changing all the time.

People with HIV or AIDS need to balance acceptance of help with preservation of control. They shouldn't give up their independence too easily, but must accept that some help is going to be necessary. They should control what they can, in small ways if it's not possible in big ways – for example, over what to wear or what to eat. But the person who is ill must remember that this level of control may be wearing for the carer. They're stuck with this situation, too, so it is important to try sharing control where possible – after all, carers have a right to eat food they like, too!

Carers should try to let the individual with HIV or AIDS determine where caring becomes smothering. People with HIV get irritated by being told solutions to problems they know are insoluble, or whose solutions only they can find – it's annoying and intrusive. General comments can be helpful: 'I'm interested in that if you want to tell me', or 'That sounds hard. How are you handling it?' If the person is crying, it is better not to try to stop them. They should be allowed to cry it out – with someone there and ready to talk if they want to. The carer should listen for cues that the person wants to talk but is afraid to be a burden or is finding it difficult to start.

It can be very hard to allow another person so much control, particularly if their illness is already taking over the carer's life. People who are feeling unwell are often cranky, and carers can end up feeling as though they have taken on a demanding and self-centred child. Or they feel manipulated and demeaned, like servants. If someone gets to the stage when they are feeling like this, they probably need some respite care – they should contact the social services department, Age Concern or the Carers National Association for advice, or some of the other support agencies listed in the Useful Addresses section.

Feelings about sex

There is no reason why people with HIV should stop having a happy, active sex life – indeed, it may be a good idea for them not to cut themselves off from the comfort of physical closeness with others, and the sense of well-being that comes from enjoying their body. Safer sex is important, of course: if one partner is not infected with HIV, they will need to be protected from it; even if both partners are positive, safer sex is recommended to protect the body's immune system from having to cope with other infections.

There are, however, many reasons why sex may become difficult for people with HIV. If they are feeling unwell, they may go off sex; if they are getting really ill or disabled, they may simply not be up to it. Some medications can reduce sex drive. Depression similarly acts as a dampener on sexual desire.

There are other reasons why sex may become problematic. Most people with HIV will have become infected through sex, and they may associate making love with getting ill. They may grieve for the carefree, unprotected sex life of the past, and see safer sex as too calculated and unspontaneous. They may feel guilty having sex at all, worried that they will pass on HIV infection. They may fear that they won't find anybody prepared to have a sexual relationship with them (if they're not currently in a relationship) or (if they are) fear their partner will abandon them for someone who doesn't have HIV. If they are starting a new sexual relationship, they may feel unsure of whether or when to disclose their HIV status – fearing that their new partner will reject them or won't respect their confidentiality.

An HIV diagnosis need not mean the end of sex. Equally, no one needs to give up sex when they pick up their bus pass. Older people with HIV may feel particularly hesitant about asking for help with sexual problems, fearing that they will be seen as disgusting or ridiculous for wanting sex 'at their age'. But we are all sexual beings and we all need intimacy, so they shouldn't be afraid to seek help from one of the organisations listed in the Useful Addresses section. In the meantime, there are other ways they can feel closeness and physical pleasure with someone else: massage, taking baths together, cuddling and so on.

Looking after emotional health should be a priority. People must value themselves and enlist sources of support – trying to communicate with them truthfully and thoughtfully. If someone is finding it very tough, they should consider counselling or therapy.

Death and beyond

When death finally comes, those left behind may experience a wide range of reactions. Common responses to bereavement include disbelief, denial, anger, relief, depression and guilt – but the truth is that there is no set pattern to this, and no timetable either. The easy assumption is that grief is felt most strongly straight after death, and then slowly ebbs away. The reality is that this is often not the case: people may feel fairly unemotional all through the funeral and for some time afterwards, and then experience intense reactions months later. So carers and other loved ones need to be prepared for bereavement as an experience that will last some time, and to plan their support accordingly.

Taking care of themselves

After a loved one has died, carers should give a high priority to looking after themselves. The experience of bereavement is very individual, and there is no right or wrong way of grieving, but people might find themselves taken aback at some of the emotions they feel.

Carers are particularly vulnerable to this: their lives have been so bound up in looking after the person with HIV that they may have all kinds of reactions to the changes facing them. It is not uncommon to feel angry with the person who has died, or relieved that at least their time is their own, or totally disorientated now they have lost their main role in life – that of a carer.

This is not helped when they are suddenly left on their own without any support. There is limited support for carers in the United Kingdom, and what help is provided is mainly there for the person who is sick. When that person dies, suddenly all the support – the home helps, the social workers, the buddies – can disappear as well, leaving the carer trying to put their life back together on their own.

Many people find it tremendously helpful to talk to others in the same position. There are some excellent voluntary organisations who can help, such as CRUSE or Compassionate Friends (for bereaved parents) or the Lesbian and Gay Bereavement Project. These are all listed in the Useful Addresses section.

If someone feels so unhappy that they just can't cope, they may need professional help from their GP or a trained counsellor. The Terrence Higgins Trust provides bereavement counselling. The GP may offer medication, and it is up to each person whether they think this is right for them or not. In the short term, anti-depressants can be very useful in helping people to get through the early days and maybe weeks. But they shouldn't use tablets as a substitute for dealing with their feelings by talking them through with someone as well.

Of course, it isn't necessary to be alone for someone to feel on their own. They may be surrounded by other grieving people and still feel totally isolated; similarly, it is easy for a person to be so wrapped up in their own grief that they become unintentionally callous about other people's. This is often the time when homosexual partners are ostracised, or when parents are frozen out of the partner's home. All the bereaved should try not to let their loss lead them to punish, blame or pull rank on other people. They should also try not to play down the extent of other people's loss compared to their own – this is particularly important with small children, who are commonly assumed to be 'too young to know what's going on' or so young that they will get over it quickly. Even very small children are affected by an atmosphere of distress, and will feel confused and unhappy at the sudden disappearance of a family member. Time must be taken to explain to them what is happening, and allow them the right to grieve too.

Bereavement need not damage relationships: it can draw people together, too, providing an opportunity for reconciliation, communication and a new understanding. Faced with the reality of a child dying, many previously estranged parents have realised the pointlessness of rejecting them while they were alive. Coming together through this crisis may inject a new honesty, urgency and warmth into family relationships. Betty has known families in which the son's partner has been a source of strength and closeness, sometimes filling the son's role after his death, and providing a second chance for loving and parenting:

❝ *I knew a young man whose parents worked abroad, while he lived in their house here with his lover. Now this nice young man died, and his parents came back from abroad to go through all the rituals and to grieve, in this house with the lover who is still there because he has nowhere else to go. They have accepted that their son was homosexual, but it did not go smoothly at first. But, you know, these parents have turned out to be wonderful. The father has now gone back abroad to work, but the mother and the young man are living there and they have a wonderful relationship. They sit together and they grieve together. But I think it's very rare that you find this* 〞

Many people who have lost loved ones through HIV and AIDS go on to help others with the disease: by buddying, counselling or providing other voluntary services. This can be an excellent idea, but care is needed to avoid taking it on as a way of healing themselves. Having experienced something does not necessarily make somebody the best person to help others in the same situation: it can be easy to assume that they are going through exactly the same experience, without seeing their individual needs and expectations. Neither should anyone fall into the trap of trying to atone for any guilt they may feel that they couldn't prevent their loved one's death by trying to 'save' others. They have nothing to feel guilty for, and their best way forward is to look after themselves first.

6.
Getting practical help

Even if people feel they can cope with their current situation, it makes sense to find out what practical support is available – for now or for the future. Some people find asking for help difficult or humiliating. The high level of unclaimed benefits by older people suggests they may see claiming as 'sponging' or being unable to support themselves, rather than as their entitlement after many years of paying National Insurance.

Similarly, some people don't like to make use of social services. They may see social workers as 'snoopers', wanting to stick their noses into everyone else's business; or they may think that only 'problem families' or 'delinquents' need social workers.

Self-sufficiency is admirable, but everyone needs help sometimes. There is nothing shameful in this: in fact, asking for and accepting just a bit of help at the right time can make it possible for people to carry on coping for longer.

If someone is caring for a person with HIV, it is important to remember that their care must be planned with them, not imposed. Being unwell can make people feel they are losing control over their own lives, and it is important that this autonomy is not further undermined by being 'taken over'. Sometimes people can seem unreasonable in their refusal to accept support services even when it is obvious than they cannot really cope. Carers must try to be patient with this: the reasons for their attitude may well be that they are scared of losing control, or determined to keep going themselves for as long as possible. Carers should by all means express their own view, but should not take control away from the person who is ill.

This is not always easy, particularly for the one being called upon to provide care that the person with HIV is refusing to allow a professional to do. One older mother provided constant care for her son, who was quite seriously ill. He refused to let anybody but her care for him – in fact, he refused to let her tell anybody about his condition, so cutting her off from the emotional support of friends as well as from the practical support of home help services. She felt she had to respect his wishes, but also felt constantly exhausted, angry and resentful.

Careful negotiation is needed to resolve this kind of situation. The loved one who is ill doesn't actually want to see their carer collapse with exhaustion, so they have a stake in finding an acceptable compromise. Reassuring them that love and commitment are not being withdrawn may help; so will serious consideration of any alternatives they may put forward. It may be helpful to bring in a respected third party to mediate, or to try any other option on a trial basis initially.

Social services

The social services department can help to organise welfare benefits, residential care, respite care and a range of help in the home. Under the NHS and Community Care Act 1990, local authorities are obliged to assess the needs of anyone who appears to need community care services – and this includes older people and people with HIV.

In order to get practical help from social services, an assessment will be carried out. The aim of this is to work out what the person's needs are and then see if services are available to meet those needs. This may involve a simple phone interview or a detailed consultation at home plus consultation with the doctor and other professionals involved – it all depends on the complexity of each case and the scale of the person's needs.

An assessment can be requested by ringing the local social services department. Different authorities have different ways of arranging assessments: some are undertaken by specialist assessors, others by social workers, occupational therapists or home care organisers. In some areas, the assessment may be carried out by an HIV Community Care Organiser.

The assessment itself is nothing to worry about. The 'assessor' will probably ask for the person's biographical details, how they currently manage their daily life, what help they may already be receiving, their income, their physical and mental health, and what kind of help they want.

Once the assessment has taken place, social services will decide what kind of help they can provide. This may include meals on wheels, bathing, home care assistants (home helps) or respite care. They must supply a written 'care plan' setting out what services will be offered. This may include what other services may be needed, and when the next assessment will take place.

The individual is usually assigned a key worker, a social worker or home care organiser, who will continue to be responsible for their care. If the situation is complex, and a lot of different people and agencies are involved, they may be assigned a care manager (also called care organiser or link worker) to co-ordinate all the different services.

As well as assessing people for help from the social services, a social worker may provide counselling, help them apply for benefits or refer them to a range of voluntary organisations to meet further needs.

Other support services

As well as social services, help might be needed from:

District nurses, who can come to a person's home to give baths, change dressings and give advice. Access through the GP.

Macmillan nursing teams, who are specially trained to care for the terminally ill, and to provide emotional as well as medical support. Access through the GP, hospital or district nurse.

Occupational therapists, whose primary task is to assess mobility in and around the home, and to arrange for the provision of aids and adaptations such as wheelchairs and bathrails. They usually work from hospitals and the social services department.

Voluntary organisations, such as Age Concern, Terrence Higgins Trust, Crossroads Care, for a wide range of services.

Counselling and self-help support, provided either through a counsellor attached to the GP surgery or hospital or through a voluntary organisation. Older people are often wary of counselling and therapy, seeing it as 'washing your dirty linen in public' or as a sign of weakness or even mental illness. This is a shame, as we all need to share our problems with someone at sometime. It is worth giving counselling a try – many people are surprised at how down-to-earth and helpful it can be.

A quick guide to support services

If someone needs . . .

Help with their daily routine

Help with housework, shopping, cleaning	*Contact social services, a voluntary organisation such as Age Concern or an AIDS agency, or a private agency*

Help with getting up, getting washed and dressed, going to the toilet, eating, getting undressed, going to bed	*Contact social services or voluntary care attendant scheme (eg Crossroads Care) or private agency*
Help with incontinence or incontinence supplies (pads, pants, bedding)	*Ask the GP to refer them to a district nurse or continence adviser*
Help with nursing, bathing, toileting, lifting	*Ask the GP to refer them to a district nurse or private nursing agency*
Help with laundry	*Social services may be able to help, but this service is increasingly vulnerable to cost-cutting. Private laundry services can be looked up in the* Yellow Pages

Help with meals

Meals on wheels	*Social services or voluntary organisations such as Age Concern, The Food Chain or Women's Royal Voluntary Service (WRVS)*
Luncheon club	*Contact social services, local community group, church or voluntary group*

Help with aids, equipment and home adaptations

Advice on equipment to help with everyday living (eg washing, cooking, using the toilet)	*Occupational therapist, via social services department or hospital*
Bedroom equipment (rails, hoist etc)	*District nurse or occupational therapist, via social services*
Mobility aids (eg wheelchair, walking sticks, walking frames)	*GP, physiotherapist or hospital*

| Short-term hire of equipment | *Local branch of British Red Cross, Age Concern or WRVS* |
| Adaptations to make their home more suitable for a disabled person | *Occupational therapist (via social services department), housing or environmental services department, or voluntary organisation* |

Help with getting about

Help with transport	*Dial-a-Ride or other voluntary organisation, social services or private taxi*
Transport to and from voluntary luncheon club, day centre etc	*Social services department or community group, or Terrence Higgins Trust 'helper cells' for hospital visits*
Transport to shops	*Community or voluntary group, Good Neighbour scheme (via social services)*
Advice about getting a specially adapted car	*Motability, Department of Social Security*
Orange parking badge	*Social services department*
Disabled Person's Railcard	*Local (staffed) railway station*

A break for the carer (respite care)

| Someone to sit with the person while the carer goes out for a few hours | *Social services department, voluntary organisation or private agency* |
| Day care in a special centre; may include lunch, social activities, use of bathing facilities, chiropody, hairdressing etc | *Social services department, hospital or voluntary organisation (eg Age Concern, London Lighthouse)* |

| Short-term care away from home, from a day to a fortnight. Could be a hospital residential home, or even with another family | *Social services department, hospital, private or voluntary residential or nursing home* |

Benefits available for people with HIV and AIDS

Claiming benefits can be a demoralising and draining experience, and this often deters people from claiming financial help that is theirs by right. Some older people still remember when claiming welfare carried a social stigma, with all the associated degradation of 'means testing'. Nevertheless, it really does make sense for people with HIV or AIDS to find out what benefits they are entitled to, because these can make all the difference to their quality of life. They can get help with claiming benefits from the social worker, or from voluntary organisations such as the Citizens Advice Bureau, Age Concern and the Terrence Higgins Trust. This should be done as early as possible, because some benefits cannot be backdated to before the first claim was made.

The financial support available varies according to each individual situation, but it is worth checking out the following.

Pensions

Someone over retirement age will probably already be receiving the basic state pension. The amount they get depends on how much National Insurance they paid while working (or while their husband was working). It is worth checking with a social worker or benefits adviser that the pension has been calculated correctly.

Benefits for carers

People of working age who cannot work full-time because of their caring responsibilities may be able to claim **Invalid Care Allowance** (ICA). This is counted as income against means-tested benefits such as Income Support or Housing Benefit; if the person with HIV is receiving the severe disability premium with Income Support, Council Tax Benefit or Housing Benefit, this will be taken off if the carer claims ICA. Seek advice on this. There is also a carer premium paid to someone who is getting Income Support, Housing Benefit or Council Tax Benefit. Carers are entitled to this if they are entitled to ICA – even if they don't get ICA because they are already getting other benefits.

Benefits for people on low incomes

Income Support tops up weekly income to a level set each year by the government. It is means-tested, and all the individual's income and savings over a certain amount will be taken into account against it. The person may also qualify for **Housing Benefit**, even if they don't qualify for Income Support. This helps with the cost of rent for people with a low income, and is claimed through the local authority. Other benefits include **Council Tax Benefit**, which is claimed in the same way as Housing Benefit. Finally, it is still worth claiming Income Support even if an individual gets only a very low payment, because it automatically opens doors to a range of other benefits, including free or reduced-cost dental treatment, prescriptions, eye tests and vouchers for glasses. People may also qualify for one-off **Social Fund** payments to help with exceptional expenses such as **Cold Weather Payments**, **Funeral Payments**, **Community Care Grants** (to help them continue living at home, or to enable them to return home from hospital) and **Crisis Loans**. Loans have to be paid back but they are interest-free.

Benefits for while someone is sick

People who are under the state pension age but too ill to work may be able to claim **Statutory Sick Pay** (SSP) (paid by the employer instead of wages for the first 28 weeks to someone too sick or disabled to work); **Incapacity Benefit** is for people who don't qualify for SSP or who have been too sick to work for over 28 weeks; **Severe Disablement Allowance** is for people who can't claim Incapacity Benefit because they haven't paid enough National Insurance. **Disability Working Allowance** is for people who are working but are on a low income because they have a disability.

People over 65 who become ill or disabled may be able to claim **Attendance Allowance**. This is paid to people who need help with personal care or need someone to watch over them. There are two rates: one for people who need care during the day only, the other for people who need attendance round the clock. This is not means-tested and doesn't affect other benefits; people applying for Attendance Allowance should usually have been disabled for six months before getting it, but if they are terminally ill they can claim straight away.

Disability Living Allowance (DLA) is for people who become disabled under the age of 65. It is made up of a 'care component', which has three levels according to how much looking after is needed, and a 'mobility component', which has two levels according to how much help is needed to get around. DLA is not means-tested and doesn't count against other benefits.

In a family with children under the age of 18, it is also worth checking other benefits such as **Family Credit, Child Benefit** and **One Parent Benefit**.

Where they live

There are a number of reasons why housing might become an important issue. Someone who has HIV will want to be sure that their home is:

- a healthy place to live – not cold or damp, for example;

- secure – so they're not always worrying about where they'll be living next;

- safe (from the threat of verbal or physical abuse from the neighbours, for example);

- accessible (if someone has a disability, they need to be able to get up the stairs, into the bath and so on);

- in a convenient location (maybe they want to live nearer the centres of excellence for HIV treatment, or nearer their family).

Carers may face the same issues if they are living in the same home. If the person with HIV or AIDS and their carer have not been living together before, they may have to consider doing so. One person moving in may present real problems if the home is too small, or if substantial changes will have to be made to the living space in order to accommodate someone else's needs.

It is easy to under-estimate how disruptive it can be to start living together. When someone moves back home after many years away, both they and their parents will have to do a lot of adjusting. It is very easy to slip back into old roles, the parents trying to control their child's life again and the child taking parental services (eg housework, cooking, offering lifts) for granted. Tensions can erupt over sensitive issues such as partners staying over, and who actually sets the house rules. The child is an adult now, and it is necessary to find a whole new way of living together.

It can also be difficult living apart, however. Carers can very quickly get worn out dashing between two homes, and there is always the worry of what might happen when they are not there. If they live at some distance, they may not be in very frequent contact: indeed, the person with HIV may have built up an 'alternative family' of partners and friends. Parents in particular can find this very painful and excluding.

So it is necessary to think through all the options very carefully. There are advantages to living alone – continued independence, familiar surroundings, less upheaval – but this may be not be an option if care needs become considerable or if loneliness is a real problem. Moving in together can be very stressful for both people, and for anybody else living in the household – it can also mean over-crowding and loss of independence. But it may provide companionship and safety, and less to-ing and fro-ing for the carer.

Housing rights

People can ask their local authority to rehouse them if they are in priority need and homeless or in unsuitable accommodation. 'Priority need' includes older people and disabled people, and may also include people with HIV. 'Unsuitable accommodation' includes housing that is overcrowded, in poor condition (cold, damp, falling apart), unsuitable for people's needs (because they cannot get up the stairs, for example) or if there is a threat of violence (perhaps from the neighbours).

Local authorities vary in their definition of what constitutes 'vulnerability', but older people are given priority. If they agree that someone needs rehousing, they may be moved into temporary accommodation until somewhere suitable is found – this will either be a council flat/house or through a housing association.

A person who is not homeless but wants to be rehoused should contact the local authority and ask to be put on their housing waiting list. Most authorities operate a 'points' system, which gives each person a higher or lower position on the waiting list according to how bad their current situation is.

Someone wanting to move to another area should contact the council's housing department in that area for advice. If there is a strong social reason for the move – for example to be nearer relatives who need caring for or who will be doing the caring – application should be made to the local authority for a move under the Homes Mobility Scheme. The individual would normally need to be a council tenant already, with quite pressing reasons for needing to move, to be speedily successful with this.

As well as trying the local authority, it may be possible to get re-housed via a housing association. Housing associations are non-profit-making organisations that provide homes for people in housing need. Some of them specialise in accommodation for older people. Information on housing associations in a chosen area is available from Age Concern England on receipt of a stamped addressed envelope.

If people are happy to stay where they are but need adaptations to make their home suitable, they may be able to claim help with doing so. The **Disabled Facilities Grant** is designed to help make a home more suitable, for example by installing a chair lift. This is a means-tested grant that is available only to people who are registered disabled. **Minor Works Grants** are available to owner occupiers or private sector tenants in receipt of Income Support, Family Credit, Housing Benefit or Council Tax Benefit. Up to £3,000 may be awarded to cover specific works such as thermal insulation. **Renovation Grants** are awarded to owner occupiers or landlords to improve accommodation deemed 'unfit for human habitation'.

Many older people opt for sheltered accommodation or residential care at this stage in their lives, and there is no reason why being HIV positive should make any difference to that. **Sheltered housing** is usually a development of 20–40 self-contained flats, with a resident scheme manager (warden) and an alarm system. Meals and personal care are not normally provided, but some organisations do provide extra support, called 'housing with care' or 'extra care sheltered housing' schemes. Some older people appreciate the extra security and the companionship of their peers in sheltered housing. Others don't like to live in a block occupied exclusively by older people, and feel cut off from their community of origin. Application for sheltered housing can be made through the local authority.

It may also be worth considering **residential** and **nursing home care**. Residential homes are for people who need help with personal care; nursing homes provide nursing care as well. These homes have had a bit of an image problem in the past, and many older people are still very worried at the prospect of giving up their independence entirely. Although it isn't always easy to find a home that meets all of an individual's requirements, most have high standards and all are regularly inspected. They can be a very good choice, providing round-the-clock care and the companionship of others. However, residential care can be very expensive, and may mean loss of independence and estrangement from family and community. It is not always easy for someone to find a home that they like and that is prepared to accept them.

Residential care can be arranged privately, if the individual can afford the fees. If people need help with the costs, they will have to be assessed by a social worker. Social services can only help with residential care fees if the person has been assessed as needing this care and being unable to live independently in the community. Their income and savings will be taken into account. Specialist advice on how to find and pay for residential care is available from voluntary organisations such as Age Concern and Counsel and Care.

Prejudice is a serious worry for older people affected by HIV, and it may be an issue with all these housing options. People with HIV can be and have been harassed by neighbours, and older people entering residential care or sheltered accommodation may be concerned that they will encounter prejudice because of their HIV status – or the HIV status of friends or relatives who may visit them. It may be necessary to seek specialist advice from one of the organisations listed at the back of this book before deciding how much should be disclosed at the time of an assessment or when viewing a residential home. Some local authorities and housing associations are very sensitive to these issues; one nursing home in west London has even organised

HIV awareness sessions for its residents, conscious that at least two of them have children with HIV or AIDS.

Medical care

Staying well

It is worth stressing again the importance of people looking after themselves even before developing symptomatic HIV disease. It can be hard to keep motivated to do this during the long months or years before symptoms develop, but it is well worth maintaining good health by getting regular medical care, following a nutritious diet, and cutting down on alcohol and smoking.

Individuals vary tremendously in how they can best keep healthy. Some prefer to keep working, while others find it less stressful to give up work and find a new pace of life. Some need to increase their level of exercise, others to make sure they get more rest. Again, the best approach for everyone is to take good medical advice and also to learn how to look after themselves – by getting informed, talking to others and listening to their own body.

It is also important for carers to look after themselves. Mothers in particular are vulnerable to sacrificing their own health for others. Carers shouldn't take on more than they can cope with, and should give themselves regular breaks and recognise if they are getting stressed so they can plan ahead. They won't be much help to anybody if they're not coping themselves.

Community-based health services

People who are HIV positive will need to organise regular medical care. The lynchpin for most healthcare provision in the United Kingdom is the **general practitioner** (GP). The GP is the key person who can refer patients to all the other health services: they will be able to give advice and treatment that is based in their knowledge of all aspects of an individual's health. A good GP is worth their weight in gold; however, a GP who seems to be uninformed or unsympathetic about HIV could be a real problem. Many people with HIV prefer to receive their regular care from **GUM clinics** (see p 20), usually the ones based in big hospitals in London and other large cities. These are centres of excellence for HIV treatment but, because of their location, they are not available to everyone.

Other community-based health services include:

district nurses, who can help with bathing, lifting, toileting, changing dressings and giving advice in the home;

health visitors, who may visit older people in their own homes and give them advice about other services;

community psychiatric nurses, who visit and advise people with mental health problems and their carers;

continence advisers, who provide advice, help and information about incontinence;

link workers, who work with people whose first language is not English.

Sometimes chiropodists, dentists and opticians will also make home visits.

It can sometimes be a struggle making sure that these community-based services provide the comprehensive, seamless care that may be needed. Social and health services are so complicated these days that it is easy to feel lost in the system, or that an individual's views and wishes are not being heard. If someone thinks they are not getting a fair deal, they should seek advice from a voluntary organisation such as Age Concern or the Terrence Higgins Trust.

Hospital and hospice care

Most people with HIV will at some stage receive hospital care, either in-patient or out-patient. Some hospitals are excellent providers of treatment for HIV and AIDS, with specially trained staff and a wealth of knowledge and great sensitivity. Unfortunately, many of these hospitals are concentrated in areas such as London and Edinburgh – where most people with HIV live. Many people with HIV have actually moved there to gain access to these services. Not everyone will feel willing to do that – and older people in particular are unlikely to want to uproot themselves from their communities and families to go hospital-chasing. The new NHS reforms, however, have given 'fundholding' GPs the power to 'buy' treatment for their patients wherever they choose. So if the GP is a fundholder, patients may be able to receive healthcare outside their own district.

When planning for or already experiencing serious illness, it is worth considering hospice care. Hospices are no longer solely places for the dying: many of them also provide respite care and short-term care for people who have been discharged from hospital but are not yet ready to return home. Hospices are also excellent providers of terminal care, with top quality pain control and emotional support, and are highly experienced in handling bereavement and follow-up care for loved ones. They usually have a much more homely atmosphere than hospitals. Some people are put off by the image of hospice care as treatment for people 'at the end of the line', unfortunately. Increasing numbers of hospices accept people with AIDS, but a number still do not for a variety of reasons.

In practice, people can and do take advantage of all these care options. For example, someone with HIV may live at home for most of their illness, using a range of community care facilities. During periods of illness they may spend time in hospital, and then choose terminal care in a hospice.

Healthcare at home

Someone with HIV or AIDS living at home may be experiencing all kinds of illnesses or none; they may be taking all kinds of medications or none; they may be on special diets or complementary medicines, or none. Whatever the individual situation, they will need medical advice on how to maximise their health at home, which includes treating the whole person and not just symptoms or illnesses as they arise. This section does not attempt to substitute for that; instead, it just takes a look at a few of the situations that may be faced and offers some ideas on how to cope better with them.

Coping with fatigue

Fatigue is a common problem for people with HIV. It may be physical or psychological in cause, and is often caused by – and contributes to – depression. Medical advice is a good idea, as some medications may help. It is important to remember, though, that the reason or reasons for depression must be addressed. Medicines may just deal with the symptoms, so it may be helpful to have counselling.

At home, people can help themselves by not taking on too much. They should try to plan their lives so that their most strenuous activities are carried out at times of the day when they tend to feel most energetic; buy healthy foods that don't need complicated preparation, or pre-prepare meals and snacks to keep in the freezer; wear clothes that don't need ironing. If they can afford it, they should get in a cleaner. 'Helper Cells' of the Terrence Higgins Trust provide all kinds of services, such as gardening, walking the dog and redecorating.

Coping with dementia

HIV-associated dementia occurs in 30–50 per cent of people with late-stage AIDS, and this incidence is probably higher among older age groups. People who have HIV, may find it a useful precaution to plan for the possible onset or worsening of dementia. They can increase their control over their own future – whether or not dementia develops – by assigning an Enduring Power of Attorney to someone they trust, writing a Living Will to establish their wishes about future medical treatment, and writing a Will to control the disposal of their assets. Advice on all these is available from Age Concern or the Terrence Higgins Trust.

They could also think through how they will decide, and when they will know, to stop certain activities. For example, at what stage will it be too risky to drive a car? When will they give up work? When will they stop living on their own?

It can be very frightening to face dementia, but in the early stages at least there is a lot that people can do to help themselves. An important principle is to plan a routine that gives the information they need at the time they need it. If someone is living on their own, they need to take particular care to remind themselves of what is happening and what they need to do next: for example, by writing lists of daily tasks and ticking them off, or leaving notes for themselves in relevant places. If the individual is living with someone else, they need to plan this together.

Caring for someone with dementia can be very stressful but there are ways in which to make the task easier. For example, people with dementia may start experiencing mental changes such as memory loss and difficulty in concentrating. They may find the following suggestions helpful:

- Memory loss can be helped by keeping an up-to-date diary, and carrying a notebook for jotting down things they will need to recall.

- Medication should be taken as directed. It is easy to forget when pills are due, so medicines should be kept in special pillboxes marked with the day and time.

- Loss of concentration is common, so lists of information should not be reeled off to someone with dementia. They should be told one thing at a time, checking that they have understood, and the information repeated later to remind them.

- A regular routine is important, and keeping a clock and calendar on display will make it easier for them to remember where they are. Moving familiar objects or redecorating unnecessarily can confuse them.

- People with dementia may grow depressed and apathetic, and lose the drive to eat, wash and generally take care of themselves. They may need to be reminded to do so, and it helps if they can be left prepared snacks and meals so that they don't have to go to the effort of cooking.

- Safety in the home must be given careful consideration. Someone with dementia may forget that they have turned the gas on, or left an iron on a heap of clothes.

- People with dementia may suffer 'motor' problems: they lose balance, their hands tremble, they drop things. Steps should be taken to make sure this is not aggravated by undetected physical problems such as failing sight or hearing difficulties.

Dementia can cause difficulties in a relationship. It is easy for carers and other loved ones to attempt to 'draw out' the person with HIV, thinking that through bright chatter and intellectual stimulation they can somehow defeat dementia. Or they may move too quickly into treating the person with HIV as a young child who cannot understand anything or work anything out for themselves. It is important to try to maintain a balance in order to preserve whatever sense of control and dignity the person with HIV has remaining.

Someone who is confused and forgetful may get argumentative, or dogmatic, when trying to assert their sense of reality. It's not helpful to go along with muddled delusions – it just confuses everyone further – but neither should carers get drawn into hopeless rows. Equally, it is helpful to continue to encourage self-esteem and independence. A person with dementia should be encouraged to do as much as they can for themselves and for the household.

When illness gets severe

Anyone caring at home for someone who is seriously ill should have received professional advice on how to look after them. Even if the person wants to die at home, the carer will still need medical support, so they should know what they are dealing with and what to expect. The carer will also need help in giving social, emotional and spiritual support. No one person can meet all the needs of another – whether they are ill or well.

Even when someone is very seriously ill, a lot can be done to make them feel happier and more comfortable. The carer can make sure they are kept clean and comfortable, turning them regularly to avoid pressure (bed) sores (the district nurse can demonstrate how to do this), keep them from getting hungry or thirsty, and make sure they have as much pain-killer as needed. They can be prevented from getting lonely by sitting with them and talking – or just by being silent, if that is what they prefer.

If the person with AIDS is up to it, this is the time to check that they have put their affairs in order. Hopefully they will have taken care of these already, but it may be necessary to make sure that they have sorted out the following.

Living Will. Also known as an advance directive, a Living Will is a statement of the person's wishes about the treatment they will want if they become too ill to express an informed choice. Living Wills are not legally binding but they do help doctors and others make their professional judgements in full knowledge of what the person would have wanted. Living Will forms are available from the Terrence Higgins Trust.

Will. A Will can reduce any uncertainty or conflict after death regarding the disposal of a dead person's estate. Again, it is far better for a Will to be made before getting seriously ill. This is particularly important for people in same-sex relationships, because the law does not recognise their legitimacy and a bereaved partner may end up with nothing.

Next of kin. A person's next of kin is the nearest blood relative(s). If a single or widowed person dies without having made a Will, the next of kin will have first claim on the estate. If an individual wants someone else to be given rights as next of kin – their partner, for example – they must say so in their Will, and tell the GP and hospital as well.

Funeral arrangements. Some people will have strong feelings about what they want to happen to them after death, and it will be important to them that they can trust their carer to honour their wishes.

The person with HIV must be the one to decide whether or not they are ready to talk about death: they should not be forced to confront death if they don't want to, but equally they should not be told comforting lies if they want to talk honestly about what is happening to them. It can be very hard for parents and carers to sit and listen to a loved one's pain and fear of death, but it is even harder for someone who knows they are dying if everyone around them keeps insisting they will get better. When the person is ready to let go, don't make them carry on fighting. It is often important to reassure a dying person that it is all right to 'move on'.

Arrangements after death

If the person with HIV has died in hospital or in a hospice, the staff there are very experienced and know the procedures. They will be able to advise about registering the death, arranging the funeral, and may also offer counselling or referral for bereavement care.

If the death has been at home, the home care team should be on hand to help. It will be necessary to call a doctor to issue a medical certificate, which is handed in when the death is registered.

A funeral director will need to be contacted, to make arrangements for burial or cremation. It is common practice for people who have died with AIDS to be sealed in a body bag, labelled 'risk of infection', and not reopened. This is an unnecessary and distressing procedure, but at the time of writing it is, unfortunately, still done by some funeral agencies.

It is possible that undertakers will be insensitive in the case of someone who has died with AIDS. It is advisable to go to an undertaker recommended by the hospital, local HIV nurse or home care team.

The person paying for the funeral may qualify for financial assistance with funeral expenses (from the Department of Social Security) if they are claiming Income Support or Housing Benefit. If there is no money available for the funeral, the local authority will organise it but it will be a very 'no frills' arrangement.

A useful booklet, which has been written with a special emphasis on AIDS, is Trevor Smith's *Before and After: Advance planning for death and funeral arrangements*, published by the Salvation Army. You may also find it helpful to consult the Benefits Agency leaflet D49 *What to do after a death*.

Where to go for information and advice: a checklist

Information about HIV and AIDS	*Terrence Higgins Trust or other AIDS charity (see 'Useful Addresses')*
Information about welfare benefits	*The Citizens Advice Bureau, welfare benefits adviser at Terrence Higgins Trust or Age Concern, local Benefits Agency (social security) office or local advice centre, or phone the Benefits Agency Freeline 0800 666555*
Information about services	*Social services department or GP*
Advice and information about adapting the home	*The occupational therapist at the social services department or Care and Repair (see 'Useful Addresses') or the renovation grants section of the local authority*
Advice about health problems	*GP, GUM clinic or consultant*
Nursing care or advice about mobility, lifting or turning someone heavy	*District nurse*
Advice about incontinence	*Continence adviser*

Information about making a Will or other legal matters	*Citizens Advice Bureau, legal adviser at Terrence Higgins Trust, law centre or solicitor*
Someone to talk to about problems	*Ask the GP for a referral to a local counsellor or community psychiatric nurse, or appropriate voluntary organisation (eg Age Concern, Carers National Association, Body Positive)*
Support in bereavement	*CRUSE, the Compassionate Friends, Lesbian and Gay Bereavement Project, Terrence Higgins Trust, Body Positive or London Lighthouse. Hospitals, hospices and churches may also offer support*
Contact with other carers	*Ask the social worker if there is a carers' group, or contact the local Council for Voluntary Service or the Carers National Association*
If someone feels desperate	*Contact the Samaritans (phone number in the local telephone directory) or the National AIDS Helpline*

A final note about HIV, AIDS and you

Whether you are an older person with HIV yourself, or a parent, grandparent, carer or friend of someone in this situation, you may find yourself at times feeling frightened and alone. There is still so much stigma and silence around this issue – particularly for older people – that it can be hard to remember that HIV is just a disease, not a curse or a judgement. In years to come, people will look back in amazement at how we treated people with HIV, just as we now look back with horror at the treatment of people with leprosy or mental illness a century ago.

But things change fast, and there is an ever-increasing amount of support available to people affected by HIV and AIDS – much of it initiated by people with HIV themselves. Many older people have been greatly helped through the challenge of AIDS by the organisations listed at the back of this book. It is still true that HIV support services are dominated by younger people – but older people can help change that by using these services themselves. It is still true that support services for older people are not generally well equipped to deal with HIV issues – but this too can be changed by older people asking for the help they need.

You can also help beat the problem by becoming part of the solution. Many older people who have encountered HIV in their own lives or in their family are now working to help others in the same situation. (As are others who have never encountered HIV themselves but who simply care and want to help.) Older people have valuable experience and time to spare, which are greatly appreciated by voluntary organisations. They are proving that AIDS is truly everybody's problem, and that everybody has a part to play in the fight against AIDS.

USEFUL ADDRESSES

Adfam National
*National helpline for the families
and friends of drug abusers, offering
confidential support and information.*

Chapel House
18 Hatton Place
London EC1N 8ND
Tel: 0171-405 3923
(10 am–5 pm
Monday–Friday)

Age Concern
See page 105 for addresses of the national headquarters.
Local branches will be listed in the telephone directory.

**AIDS Care Education and
Training (ACET)**
*A church-based organisation that gives
practical help to people with AIDS,
including home care and grants to help
with household bills, equipment
and holidays.*

PO Box 3693
London SW15 2BQ
Tel: 0181-780 0400

AIDS Helpline Northern Ireland
*Free advice and information on HIV
and AIDS.*

Tel: 01232 326117

Bethany
*Offers rest and respite care for people
with HIV and AIDS.*

St Mary's Road
Bodmin
Cornwall PL31 1NF
Tel: 01208 79035

Black HIV–AIDS Network (BHAN)

Provides support for black people with HIV or AIDS, and black people working in the field.

1st Floor
St Stephen's House
41 Uxbridge Road
London W12 8LH
Tel: 0181-749 2828

Blackliners

Provide HIV and AIDS information to black and Asian communities, including leaflets, posters, counselling and support groups.

Eurolink Business Centre
49 Effra Road
London SW2 1BZ
Tel: 0171-738 5274

Body Positive

Services and support by and for people with HIV. The London office provides a range of services, including a drop-in centre, advice sessions, counselling and therapy, and a newsletter. It also provides information on regional Body Positive groups throughout the UK.

51b Philbeach Gardens
London SW5 9EB
Tel: 0171-835 1045
(Centre)
Tel: 0171-373 9124
(Helpline)

British Association for Counselling

Can give information about counselling services in your area.

1 Regent Place
Rugby
Warwickshire CV21 2PJ
Tel: 0178-857 8328/9

CARA (Care and Resources for People Affected by AIDS–HIV)

Works to develop the church response to HIV and AIDS, and provides spiritual, emotional and practical support to people with HIV or AIDS and their families and friends.

The Basement
178 Lancaster Road
London W11 1QU
Tel: 0171-792 8299

Cardiff AIDS Helpline

Free advice and information on HIV and AIDS

PO Box 304
Cardiff CF2 4NE
Tel: 01222 223443

Care and Repair
Advice about home repairs and improvements.

Castle House
Kirtley Drive
Nottingham NG7 1LD
Tel: 0115-979 9091

Carers National Association
Provides support to carers across the UK, and campaigns on their behalf. Local groups across the UK.

20–25 Glasshouse Yard
London EC1A 4JS
Tel: 0171-490 8818
0171-490 8898
(Adviceline, 1–4 pm weekdays)

Catholic AIDS Link
Spiritual, emotional and practical support to those affected by HIV or AIDS, and training, counselling and networking facilities for staff.

PO Box 646
London E9 6QP
Tel: 0171-485 7298

Citizens Advice Bureau
Free advice on legal, financial and consumer matters. Branches across the UK: your local bureau will be listed in Yellow Pages *under 'Counselling and advice'.*

Compassionate Friends
Provides support and comfort to bereaved parents.

53 North Street
Bristol BS3 1EN
Tel: 0117-953 9639

Councils for Voluntary Service (CVS)
Branches in most cities and large towns. They may be able to offer a range of voluntary services themselves or refer you to an appropriate provider. Look them up in the telephone directory or ask at your local library or Citizens Advice Bureau.

Counsel and Care
Provides advice for older people and their families.

Lower Ground Floor
Twyman House
16 Bonny Street
London NW1 9PG
Tel: 0171-485 1566

Crossroads Care
Operates a home care attendant scheme.

10 Regent Place
Rugby
Warwickshire CV21 2PN
Tel: 0178-857 3653

CRUSE – Bereavement Care
Network of bereavement support groups across the UK.

Cruse House
126 Sheen Road
Richmond
Surrey TW9 1UR
Tel: 0181-940 4818

Department of Social Security (DSS)
Free information on welfare benefits.

Tel: Freephone
0800 666555

FFLAG (Families and Friends of Lesbians and Gays)
A national organisation providing confidential support for parents and their gay, lesbian or bisexual sons or daughters, and their friends.

PO Box 153
Manchester M60 1LP
Tel: 0161-628 7621
(9 am–9 pm)
0153-370 8331
(9 am–9 pm)

The Food Chain
The Food Chain delivers a weekly Sunday three-course meal to people with AIDS in the Greater London area.

c/o BM Food Chain
London WC1N 3XX
Tel: 0181-801 4286

Grandma's
Free and confidential advice and practical help for children affected by HIV and AIDS, their parents and carers.

PO Box 1392
London SW6 4EJ
Tel: 0171-610 3904

The Griffin Project
A continuing care project for people with HIV infection and a history of drug use. It provides respite, convalescent and palliative care and drug management.

6 Penywern Road
London SW5 9ST
Tel: 0171-373 9826

Haemophilia Society
Information, advice and support for people with haemophilia and their families.

123 Westminster Bridge Road
London SE1 7HR
Tel: 0171-928 2020

Help the Aged
Works to improve the quality of life for older people by identifying needs and developing aid programmes.

16–18 St James's Walk
London EC1R OBE
Tel: 0171-253 0253
0800 289494 (Seniorline)

Hospice Information Service
Information about local hospices, which care for people who are terminally ill.

St Christopher's Hospice
51–59 Lawrie Park Road
London SE26 6DZ
Tel: 0181-778 9252

The Landmark
Day centre for people with HIV and AIDS, with services including nursing, massage, acupuncture, transport and social work support.

47 Tulse Hill
London SW2 2TN
Tel: 0181-678 6686

LEAN (London East AIDS Network)
Voluntary group that provides support services for people with HIV in east London, including small grants and information in Asian languages.

35 Romford Road
London E15 4LY
Tel: 0181-519 9545

Lesbian and Gay Bereavement Project
Counselling, advice and support for lesbians, gay men, and their families and friends.

Vaughan M Williams Centre
Colindale Hospital
London NW9 5HG
Tel: 0181-200 0511
(3–6 pm weekdays)
Tel: 0181-455 8894
(7 pm–midnight)

**London Lesbian and
Gay Switchboard**
*24-hour service offering confidential
advice and information to lesbians and
gays, their families and friends, both in
London and throughout the UK.*

BM Switchboard
PO Box 7324
London N1 9QS
Tel: 0171-837 7324

London Lighthouse
*Range of services, including residential
care, day centre, drop-in, counselling,
support groups, complementary
therapies, counselling, information
and outreach home support.*

111–117 Lancaster Road
London W11 1QT
Tel: 0171-792 1200

Mainliners
*Services for drug users and ex-drug
users with HIV or with concerns about
HIV and AIDS, including helpline,
counselling, advice and information.*

205 Stockwell Road
London SW9 9SL
Tel: 0171-738 4656

Mildmay Mission Hospital
*Independent, Christian charitable
hospital for people with AIDS.
Specialist AIDS hospice unit and
continuing care unit providing respite,
rehabilitative, convalescent and
terminal care. Counselling support,
day care and home care back-up
also available.*

Hackney Road
London E2 7NA
Tel: 0171-739 2331

Milestone House
*Continuing care unit for people
living in the Lothian area. Respite,
convalescent and palliative care.*

113 Oxgangs Road North
Edinburgh EH14 1EB
Tel: 0131-441 6989

Motability
Cars and wheelchairs for disabled people.

2nd Floor
Gate House
Westgate
Harlow
Essex CM20 1HR
Tel: 0127-963 5666

National AIDS Helpline
Free advice and information on any aspect of HIV and AIDS.
0800 567123 (24 hours)
0800 282445 (Asian languages 6 pm–10 pm Wednesdays)
0800 282446 (Cantonese 6 pm–10 pm Wednesdays)
0800 282447 (Arabic 6 pm–10 pm Wednesdays)
0800 521361 (Minicom for deaf/hard of hearing 10 am–10 pm daily)
0800 555777 (Health Literature Line 24 hours)

National Association of Bereavement Services
Information about bereavement and loss counselling services in your area.

20 Norton Folgate
London E1 6DB
Tel: 0171-247 1080
(24-hour answerphone)

National Drugs Helpline
Free 24-hour advice and information on any aspect of drug use.

Tel: 0800 776600

Patrick House
A residential home for people with brain impairment related to HIV and AIDS.

17 Rivercourt Road
London W6 9LD
Tel: 0181-846 9117

Positive Options
Help and support for families affected by HIV and AIDS.

354 Goswell Road
London EC1V 7LQ
Tel: 0171-278 5039

Positive Partners
Self-help group for people affected by HIV, including partners, families and carers. Services include support groups, counselling, complementary and alternative therapies, advice and small grants.

The Annex
Jan Rebane Centre
12–14 Thornton Street
London SW9 0BL
Tel: 0171-738 7333

Positively Children
Group set up under the auspices of Positive Partners for people with HIV aged under 18, or who have a parent or guardian with HIV, and also for parents of children with HIV and AIDS.

The Annex
Jan Rebane Centre
12–14 Thornton Street
London SW9 0BL
Tel: 0171-738 7333

Positively Irish Action on AIDS
Advice and support for Irish people affected by HIV and AIDS.

St Margaret's House
21 Old Ford Road
London E2 9PL
Tel: 0181-983 0192

Positively Women
Wide range of counselling and support services for women with HIV and AIDS.

5 Sebastian Street
London EC1V 0HE
Tel: 0171-490 5515

RADAR (Royal Association for Disability and Rehabilitation)
Information about aids and mobility, holidays, sport and leisure for disabled people,

12 City Forum
250 City Road
London EC1V 8AF
Tel: 0171-250 3222

The Red Admiral Project
Counselling and support for people with HIV, their partners, family and friends.

51a Philbeach Gardens
London SW5 9EB
Tel: 0171-835 1495

Relatives Association
Support and advice for the relatives of people in a residential or nursing home or hospital long-term.

5 Tavistock Place
London WC1H 9SN
Tel: 0171-916 6055

Samaritans   Tel: 0171-734 2800
Someone to talk to if you are in despair.
Local branches across the UK – look up
in the telephone directory.

Scottish AIDS Monitor
Information and advice about HIV and AIDS.

EDINBURGH BRANCH   GLASGOW BRANCH
26 Anderson Place   22 Woodside Terrace
Edinburgh EH6 5NP   Glasgow G3 7XH
Tel: 0131-555 4850   Tel: 0141-353 3133

Standing Conference of Ethnic   5 Westminster Bridge Road
Minority Senior Citizens   London SE1 7XW
Information, support and advice for   Tel: 0171-928 0095
older people from ethnic minorities and
their families.

The Sussex Beacon   Bevendean Road
Continuing care unit for people with   Brighton BN2 4DE
HIV and AIDS, offering respite,   Tel: 0173 694222
convalescent and palliative care.

The Terrence Higgins Trust   52–54 Grays Inn Road
Largest HIV and AIDS charity in UK,   London WC1X 8JU
with services including helpline,   Tel: 0171-831 0330
buddying, counselling, legal helpline,   0171-242 1010 (Helpline)
welfare advice, hardship grants, prison   0171-405 2381 (Legal Line)
visits and support groups

Women's Royal Voluntary Service   234–244 Stockwell Road
(WRVS)   London SW9 9SP
Provides meals at home for ill and   Tel: 0171-416 0146
disabled people in some areas.

FURTHER READING

Publications on HIV and AIDS

HIV & AIDS affects older people too
Leaflet by AIDS Concern and Education for the Over 50s.

HIV? AIDS? We're older people – it's not our problem!
HIV? AIDS? We're older gay men – its not a problem!
Leaflets by Age Concern.

Are you over 50 years old?
HIV, AIDS and Older People
Does someone you care about have AIDS?
Leaflets by Age Concern.

These leaflets are obtainable from the Services Department Unit,
Age Concern England, 1268 London Road, London SW16 4ER.

A Crisis of Silence: HIV, AIDS and Older People
Tara Kaufmann, Age Concern London, 1993.

A Time to Lie? Older People, HIV and Housing
AIDS and Housing Project, 1994.
Available from the AIDS and Housing Project,
16–18 Strutton Ground, London SW1P 2HP. Tel: 0171-222 6933.

When somebody dies

Before and After: Advance planning for death and funeral arrangements
Trevor Smith, published by the Salvation Army.

What to do after a death
Benefits Agency leaflet D 49.

Other useful publications

See pages 106–108 for details of other useful publications, published by Age Concern England.

ABOUT AGE CONCERN

HIV & AIDS and older people is one of a wide range of publications produced by Age Concern England, the National Council on Ageing. Age Concern England is actively engaged in training, information provision, fundraising and campaigning for retired people and those who work with them, and also in the provision of products and services such as insurance for older people.

A network of over 1,400 local Age Concern groups, with the support of around 250,000 volunteers, aims to improve the quality of life for older people and develop services appropriate to local needs and resources. These include advice and information, day care, visiting services, transport schemes, clubs, and specialist facilities for older people who are physically and mentally frail.

Age Concern England is a registered charity dependent on public support for the continuation and development of its work.

Age Concern England
1268 London Road
London SW16 4ER
Tel: 0181-679 8000

Age Concern Scotland
113 Rose Street
Edinburgh EH2 3DT
Tel: 01222 371566

Age Concern Cymru
4th Floor
1 Cathedral Road
Cardiff CF1 9SD
Tel: 0131-220 3345

Age Concern Northern Ireland
3 Lower Crescent
Belfast BT7 1NR
Tel: 01232 245729

Publications from ♦♠♣ Books

A wide range of titles is published by Age Concern England under the ACE Books imprint.

Health and care

Caring in a Crisis: What to do and who to turn to

Marina Lewycka

At some point in their lives millions of people find themselves suddenly responsible for organising the care of an older person with a health crisis. Very often such carers have no idea what services are available or who can be asked for support. This book is designed to act as a first point of reference in just such an emergency, signposting readers on to many more detailed, local sources of advice.

£6.95   0–86242–166–7

Caring in a Crisis: Caring for someone who is dying

Penny Mares

Confronting the knowledge that a loved one is going to die soon is always a moment of crisis. And the pain of the news can be compounded by the need to take responsibility for the care and support given in the last months and weeks. This book attempts to help readers cope with their emotions, identify the needs which the situation creates and make the practical arrangements necessary to ensure that the passage through the period is as smooth as possible.

£6.95   0–86242–158–6

Vitality and Virility: A guide to sexual health for men in mid-life

Neil Davidson

Many men in mid-life notice a decline in their physical energy, perceive this as a threat to their masculinity – particularly with regard to sexual performance and attraction – and consequently feel diminished. This book examines the truth behind the so-called 'male menopause' and addresses in practical terms many of the sexual and relationship issues which cause concern.

£7.95   0–86242–137–3

Healthy Eating on a Budget

Sara Lewis and Dr Juliet Gray

Eating a healthy, nutritionally balanced diet is important for everyone, especially older people, who often have particular health concerns. Yet for many older people their restricted budget means that choice often has to take second place to cost. The book contains over 100 carefully costed recipes, all of which are flagged up to highlight their nutritional value and their calorie content. Using these recipes, two people can eat well for a week for just over £30, without sacrificing taste or variety.

£6.95   0–86242–170–5

Money Matters

Your Rights 1995–96

Sally West

A highly acclaimed annual guide to the State benefits available to older people. Includes current information on Income Support, Housing Benefit and retirement pensions, and provides advice on how to claim them.

£3.25   0–86242–178–0

Managing Other People's Money

Penny Letts

Foreword by the Master of The Court of Protection

The management of money and property is usually a personal and private matter. However, there may come a time when someone else has to take over on either a temporary or a permanent basis. This book looks in detail at those circumstances and provides a step-by-step guide to the arrangements which have to be made.

£5.95   0-86242-090-3

If you would like to order any of these titles, please write to the address below, enclosing a cheque or money order for the appropriate amount made payable to Age Concern England. Credit card orders may be made on 0181-679 8000.

Mail Order Unit
Age Concern England
PO Box 9
London SW16 4EX

Information factsheets

Age Concern England produces over 30 factsheets on a variety of subjects. Among these the following titles may be of interest to readers of this book:

Factsheet 7 *Making your Will*

Factsheet 18 *A brief guide to money benefits*

Factsheet 23 *Help with incontinence*

Factsheet 27 *Arranging a funeral*

To order factsheets

Single copies are available free on receipt of a 9" × 6" sae. If you require a selection of factsheets or multiple copies totalling more than five, charges will be given on request.

A complete set of factsheets is available in a ring binder at a cost of £36, which includes the first year's subscription. The current cost for annual subscription for subsequent years is £17. There are different rates of subscription for people living outside the UK.

INDEX

ADDENDUM   APRIL 1996

HIV & AIDS and older people

The Carers (Recognition and Services) Act 1995 became law
from 1 April 1996. If you are providing a substantial amount
of care to someone on a regular basis, from 1 April 1996 you
have the right to ask the local authority to also consider
your needs when they are assessing the needs of the person
for whom you care.